The Good Book of

Godliness

Jack H. McQuaig

Order this book online at www.trafford.com
or email orders@trafford.com

Most Trafford titles are also available at major online book retailers.

Printed in Victoria, BC, Canada.

ISBN: 978-1-4269-1948-0 (soft)
ISBN: 978-1-4269-1949-7 (hard)

Library of Congress Control Number: 2009940291

Our mission is to efficiently provide the world's finest, most comprehensive book publishing service, enabling every author to experience success. To find out how to publish your book, your way, and have it available worldwide, visit us online at www.trafford.com

Trafford rev. 7/30/2010

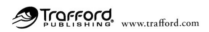 www.trafford.com

North America & international
toll-free: 1 888 232 4444 (USA & Canada)
phone: 250 383 6864 ♦ fax: 812 355 4082

Biography
Jack H. McQuaig

Jack McQuaig has spent his life helping people to find their goals and achieve them. As an Industrial Psychologist, he has advised management in organizations of all sizes how to bring better methods of hiring and training into their businesses.

He is the author of ten books on management and physical and mental fitness and his concern has always been to help people to be more effective at their work. A master's degree in psychology and a lifetime of appraising and motivating personnel have given him insight into what makes people happy and successful.

Since his semi-retirement, he has turned to the study of spirituality to find happiness and peace of mind. His conclusion is that achieving material things, gaining power and developing skills do not give all the answers to the most important things in life.

Table of Contents

Also by Jack H. McQuaig

How to Pick Men
Frederick Fell Inc.

How to Motivate Men
Frederick Fell Inc.

How to Interview and Hire Productive People
(with Peter L. and Donald H. McQuaig)
Frederick Fell Inc.

Challenge Yourself and Live
General Publishing

Your Business, Your Son and You
B. Kein Publications

The Pregnant Male
Hunter Carlyle Publishing

Synergy and the Power of Personal Proficiency
Hunter Carlyle Publishing

Like Yourself and Live
Hunter Carlyle Publishing

On the Path to Spiritual Fitness
Hunter Carlyle Publishing

Improve Your Golf with Spirituality
Hunter Carlyle Publishing

Yes, You Can Quit Smoking
Hunter Carlyle Publishing

Eustress – the Secret of Happiness and Success
Hunter Carlyle Publishing

Lunch with the Boss
Hunter Carlyle Publishing

Introduction

Why am I writing another book? Because I have created a religion called Godliness and every religion should have a Bible. I can't write a Bible so I have to settle for a book.

I will try to write a powerful book so that the followers of Godliness will have a super book to support them.

This book will give anyone who has a problem some good advice on how to cope with it. I want this book to be helpful to anyone who reads it.

The advice will be profound and valid not because of my knowledge and understanding but because of the information that comes from the super women and men who wrote the books, magazine articles and made the speeches which were the sources of my material.

I will attempt to pass along to the readers of this book the knowledge of the world's greatest thinkers.

In the religion of Godliness all I need is God. The God of my religion is caring, and filled with unconditional love.

In the religion of Godliness there is no heaven or hell. God doesn't punish you. He loves you unconditionally. If you do something wrong he will counsel you and help you to correct your ways.

In Godliness there are no commandments. God doesn't command you. He teaches you not to command others so why would he command you?

All God expects of you is that you help others and contribute something to any situation in which you are involved.

This is how the Godliness believer thinks and acts:

1. God is running the world. I don't resist. I follow his will.

2. The world is operating perfectly.

3. God is always within me and the power of the universe is flowing through me

4. We are all connected

5. Try to help others where possible

6. Try to contribute something to any situation in which you are involved.

7. You have unconditional love for everyone

8. You are controlled by the pictures in your mind. Visualize what you want and it will happen

9. Listen to your intuition and check it out

10. Welcome adversities. You learn more from them than from anything else

11. Believe everybody loves you and is trying to help you

12. You are a spirit in a body

13. The present is very important, try to stay in it

14. You are part of a great intelligent system and you are here for the purpose of helping others

15. Everything happens for a reason. There are no coincidences

16. There is a spiritual solution to every problem

17. Happiness will be your natural state if you visualize it

18. Stop thinking of yourself and start thinking of others if you want to be happy

19. Laugh and smile and you will be happy

20. You are a perfect spirit who is running your body

21. You are given a perfect body to help you through the world. Look after it

22. Connect with your fellow men one on one or in groups as much as possible. This will help you to be healthy and happy

23. Exercise your mind as well as your body

24. Have a constant physical challenge with an exercise program which will keep you in good physical condition

25. Get a mental challenge by reading good books, taking courses, talking with intelligent people and writing books

Chapter One

Affirm

Affirmations are positive thoughts on which you concentrate to achieve your goals. These thoughts can change your attitudes and alter your beliefs and get eustress working for you. Affirmations help you to communicate your ambitions and attitudes to your subconscious mind. For example, you might use this affirmation,

**"God is always with me, loving
me, caring for me and guiding me.
Thank you God, I love you God."**

You will be able to bring yourself into the spiritual orbit and have the belief that God is always with you, by using affirmations.

Affirmations can reach into your subconscious mind to get it cooperating with you to activate eustress which is the stress you get when something good happens to you. The subconscious is

Chapter One
Affirm

powerful and has a great influence on your behavior and attitudes. It is important to get your subconscious working for you.

You can use affirmations to change your attitudes or to change your actions. You can create an affirmation to help you to eliminate distress and improve yourself. There are books, which will give you suggested affirmations. Two of these are, Words that Heal, by Douglas Block, Bantam Books, and, What to Say When You Talk to Yourself, by Shad Helmstetter, Pocket Books.

You can create your own affirmations. Keep trying until you get an affirmation that feels just right.

**"God is always with me, loving
me, caring for me and guiding me.
Thank you God, I love you God,"**

It took me time and many repetitions until I felt this affirmation was just right. However, it may not be right for you. Work at it until you find some wording that activates positive thinking for you.

There are a few things to consider about an affirmation if you want it to help you to relieve distress. First, it should be positive. Negative affirmations don't work. For example, if you are trying to reduce your weight, don't make an affirmation to get rid of a

Chapter One
Affirm

certain number of pounds. Rather make the affirmation positive. It could be,

"I am looking slim and healthy."

Second, you should always have your affirmations in the present. Don't make it,

"I am going to look slim and healthy,

but rather,

"I am looking slim and healthy."

An important factor to consider in using affirmations is that repetition helps. Keep saying it over and over during the day or when you are going to sleep at night or when you waken in the morning. Can you make it rhyme? Can you say it louder or with feeling? Can you chant it? Can you sing it? Can you visualize it happening when you repeat it? These techniques can be helpful in getting an affirmation that works. You can also make your affirmation more effective by including a thank you as I have done in this affirmation,

Chapter One
Affirm

**"God is always with me, loving
me, caring for me and guiding me.
Thank you God, I love you God."**

Another way to strengthen your affirmation is to write it down. Make copies of it to put in prominent places such as, on your bedroom wall, or in your car. In this way, you will constantly visualize it. I believe there is an affirmation that will help you to relieve distress. It may take some work to find it. Keep experimenting. Make changes until you feel comfortable with your affirmation and until you feel it is working.

Don't expect magic. Certain attitudes and ideas have been with you for a long time. If you have had a bad attitude about something for ten years maybe you should be satisfied to correct it in ten years with the right affirmation. I don't believe it will be this slow to work. If it isn't bringing you the results you want, try a completely new affirmation.

The best example I can give you of how affirmations work is an experience I had. At one time I was very fearful, afraid of dying, afraid of getting sick, afraid of losing my energy and afraid of practically everything. A friend of mine suggested that I had to get rid of these fears or they would cause me much distress. I agreed.

Chapter One
Affirm

Because of these fears I made up an affirmation, which I repeated constantly in my meditation and chanting sessions. The affirmation was,

"I am brave, I am courageous, I am fearless because God is always with me."

I kept repeating this affirmation, morning, noon and night. Gradually, my fear disappeared and I became stronger.

These methods are simple and easy to use and practice has helped me stay focused on getting what I want.

The most powerful affirmations are short and to the point. Choose affirmations that seem right for you. Choose something in which you believe and which you feel you can bring into reality.

If you can bring God into your affirmation that will give it more strength. For example "God is always helping me to be happy" should be effective.

Act happy – if you want to be happy act as if you are happy. Affirm that you are happy by constantly repeating "I am happy, I am happy. If you move and think you are happy, you will become happy.

The Good Book of Godliness
Notes

Chapter Two

Believe

Your beliefs can keep you younger. If you believe, you can live to an advanced age, you probably will.

I am ninety-four years of age partly because I read a book "How to be always well", by Dr. Robert Jackson, a Canadian Medical doctor. When I was 21 years of age this book gave me the formula for living to an advanced age. I believed that I could do it by following his system of exercising and dieting and it worked.

There's a statement made by the late Norman Cousins, "Belief creates biology."

Dr. Norman Cousins proved that his beliefs were so powerful that he could survive when several doctors told him that he would die from his incurable disease within a year.

Chapter Two
Believe

Strong beliefs enabled Dr.Cousins to survive by following his program of positive thinking and acting. Not only did he survive but he was able to become a successful University Professor teaching doctors how believing could help people to keep healthy. He has spelled out his philosophy of positive thinking in his book *Head First: The Biology of Hope and the Healing Power of the Human Spirit by Penguin Books.*

Beliefs in the positive have helped me and I know they can help you to achieve your goals.

Try to believe in something. John Stuart Mill once wrote: "One person with a belief is equal to a force of ninety-nine who are only interested." A belief is a faith and an attitude that can give you meaning and purpose in your life. Beliefs change your state and give you the energy to take action and attain your goals.

The ultimate strength is to believe in God. To do this, you must concentrate on your internal life and derive your strength from knowing you are connected with an Internal Strength that is giving you the energy to survive in the external world. This doesn't' mean you have to become an introverted person and cut yourself off from enjoying the external world.

You can socialize and be active in situations involving others, but you will always be aware that you are being supported in

Chapter Two
Believe

everything you do by a Super Internal Power. This will give you great strength. If you keep your contact alive with the Great Universal Power, you will be able to go through life feeling good.

If you believe you can, you will be able to face the reverses, turn downs and resistances of life without losing control or becoming depressed. You will know that you are supported and backed up by something that is all knowing and all powerful. What courage and energy this will give you in your day to day activities! However, to do this is not easy because the stresses and pressures of day to day living are immediate and demanding. It will take discipline and concentration to keep connected with your Super Power when you are faced with constant demands from your environment. You must develop the habit of tapping this Inner Strength. One way to do this is to close your eyes from time to time and block out the present stresses by thinking of the Internal Powerhouse to which you have access. You could eventually open yourself to believing that there is a God out there in the universe willing to back you up in everything you are trying to do. With this unlimited strength at your disposal, you can certainly achieve your maximum in the outer world.

A belief is a system or a principle that provides meaning and guidance in your life. If you believe in something, your brain will tend to screen out any ideas or thoughts that do not conform to

Chapter Two
Believe

your belief. Your brain does what it is told, and a belief is a direct communication to your brain. If you believe in something, your brain will try to make it happen.

For example, in medical experiments when people are told that a certain capsule will cure a headache, a high percentage of people who take the capsule will have their headaches cured although the capsule only contains water. The belief is so strong that it executes a curing effect.

If you believe that you can achieve something, the chances are good that you will do it. On the other hand, if you believe you can't do something, you will likely fail when you try. When you believe something with all your heart and soul, you are giving an order to your subconscious mind to carry it out.

Probably more people are held back from achieving their goals by lack of belief in themselves than for any other reason. Personally, I know I could have started to write books twenty years sooner in my life if I had believed that I could do it. I had excellent ideas for two books twenty years before Iwrote them. Why didn't I take some action and write, which I really wanted to do? Because I didn't believe in myself. I had low self-esteem. My attitude was that you had to have great talent and creativity to write a book neither of which I thought I had.

Chapter Two
Believe

Twenty years later Frederick Fell, a New York publisher, was in my audience when I was speaking to a group of sales executives in New York on "How to Pick Winners". Fell approached me after my speech and said, "You could write a book on this." My answer was that I would love to write a book but I lacked the talent. What I really lacked was belief in myself.

Frederick Fell changed my beliefs about myself. I started to believe that I could write the book and I did. It was published by his company in New York in 1962 under the title How to Pick Men. If Frederick Fell hadn't changed my beliefs, I would never have written a book.

The best way to change your beliefs about yourself is to visualize what you want to believe and let your subconscious mind work on it. For example, supposing you are a taxi driver who wants to become a teacher but you don't believe that you have the leadership ability or the mature attitudes needed to teach others. Let's assume that you have a high school education. Although you have the intelligence, you lack self-esteem. You don't believe you are a worthwhile person.

You can change that belief by visualizing yourself going to night school to get a university degree. See yourself becoming more confident and developing more self-esteem. See yourself graduating in five years. Hear what the university president is

Chapter Two
Believe

saying. See it, hear it, feel it. Turn up the brightness, focus and colors to make it more compelling. Want it to happen, believe it will happen, expect it will happen and it will happen.

Your subconscious mind will now start to move you in the direction indicated by the pictures in your mind. Your beliefs will change and you will start to feel that you can do it. Your subconscious mind will show you the way and you will soon be getting suggestions to take actions that will move you closer to your outcome.

Limiting beliefs are one of the greatest obstacles to feeling good. You will not be able to feel good until you believe you can. Once this blockage has been removed and you are giving your subconscious mind new, positive messages, it will start to act on them and you will start to feel good.

The message is clear. Decide what you want to do regardless of whether you believe you can do it or not. Visualize yourself doing it. Notice how you feel, and leave it to your subconscious mind to show you the way. When you get the signal to do something, take action and your beliefs will change and work to help you to get the results you want.

In addition to having certain beliefs in life that will guide you, it is important for you to know what your values are.

Chapter Two
Believe

Values are the more personal aspect of your belief system. You can believe that everything happens for the best, have respect for people, take responsibility for your behavior, and persist until you get results, but you may still not be happy because you have the wrong results.

Your values are your beliefs about what is right and wrong for you and about who you are and what your goals should be. If you aren't doing what you think is right, you will suffer dissatisfaction and frustration. When you are doing what conforms to your values, you will be happy and feel good.

It's important to have your daily work in the field of your highest values, otherwise you will be dissatisfied. If your job is in the area of your highest values, you will be enthusiastic and will probably perform in an excellent manner.

In any relationship you have with people, it is vital to know the values of those involved. Many conflicts are caused because one person doesn't respect the values of another person. For example, if one person in a marriage is a spender and the other person is a saver, these different values will cause some conflicts. If one is sociable and the other is unsociable, there will be problems working out a satisfactory relationship. The best relationships are those in which people have the same values.

Chapter Two
Believe

The values that are most important to you are the keys to your success and happiness. For example, you could make a million in business and yet be miserably unhappy if your values indicate that you want to spend your time thinking and philosophizing and helping people with their problems rather than accumulating wealth and the things you can buy with it.

Every person has a set of values, which are really their personal philosophy of what life is all about. So let's take a look at some values and see which things are most important to you and will make you feel good.

I am going to give you a list of the things most people want, the things they value in life. Everybody wants all these things and this makes us all alike. But each person wants a different combination of these things and this makes us all different.

Which of these items is most important to you? Try to rate them for yourself from one to twenty-five. In doing this, assume that you are going to have a moderate amount of all these things in your life but the ones you rate highest will have above average amounts of that particular quality. For example, if you rate freedom and independence as number one it means that this is exceptionally important to you and you want complete independence.

Chapter Two
Believe

Here is a list of my values:

1. Money or material things
2. Security
3. Efficiency
4. Helping others
5. Health
6. Self-esteem
7. The esteem of others
8. Creativity
9. Freedom and independence
10. Sociability
11. Success
12. Opportunity
13. Health
14. Thinking and philosophizing
15. Peace of mind
16. Power
17. Honesty
18. Loyalty
19. Team work
20. Love
21. Family
22. Sex
23. Companionship
24. Peace of Mind
25. Physical Activity

By going over this list of values, you can approximately determine the type of career you should follow. For example, I want all of these things but above all I want freedom and independence. That's probably why I chose to go into business for myself. I hate to be supervised or managed by anyone else.

My next choice would be to have exceptional health, because I believe with really good health you can do almost anything you want to do. That's probably why I am in the field of mental health.

Chapter Two
Believe

My third choice would be peace of mind. What value is money or fame if you don't feel good about it?

My fourth choices would be family. Your family is the greatest source of satisfaction you can have.

My fifth choice would be to help others. All my work and writing is in the area of helping others with their problems.

My sixth choice would be money because I think it gives me more alternatives and the freedom to live as I want and avoid doing routine kinds of work.

My seventh choice would be to have others think well of me. I like recognition and this may have directed me into the public-speaking and seminar-giving fields and into the writing of books.

Number eight to me would be satisfaction from achievement. I like to enjoy what I am doing and l want to get a feeling of accomplishment from learning or developing skills.

My recommendation is that you go over this list and pick out your number one choice as a value. Compare it with each of the other twenty-four values to make sure nothing else surpasses your choice. Next pick your number two choice and compare it with the remaining twenty-three choices to make sure it stands up as number two.

Chapter Two
Believe

Keep choosing until you have selected your top eight choices and then try to fashion your career and hobbies in areas supported by your strongest values. It's important to believe in what you are doing, and only when you are working and playing in the fields of your values will you be happy and feel good.

Your attitudes are formed by your beliefs and values and all of your attitudes form your philosophy of living. The purpose of having a powerful philosophy of life is to enable you to feel good about yourself and others and about life in general. To do this you must be happy and get real satisfaction from living. One of the best ways to do this is to enjoy the simple things in life: walking in the country, reading an interesting book, eating a good meal, sunbathing, watching a good movie or an interesting television show, listening to your favorite music or talking to a friend.

These are among the most pleasant experiences in the world and yet all of these things are available to practically everyone. Large amounts of money are not required to do these things. Nor is great intelligence or education needed. To enjoy the simple things in life which are always available, it is vital to be in a good mental state. So start to appreciate the basic things in life and enjoy them as much as you can right now. Plan for the future but live for the present. I've noticed that really happy people not only enjoy the simple pleasures but relish them and build them into their lives.

Chapter Two
Believe

I got a great lesson in this a few years ago when I was driving three handicapped children home from a Christmas party that our Rotary Club had given for handicapped children. The three kids lived in relative poverty in addition to having severe handicaps. However, on the way home from the party these three children broke out singing Christmas carols. They were getting satisfaction from the simple things in life and were enjoying the present. They were not worrying about the life of poverty to which they were soon to return and the extreme handicaps they would carry with them for life. This was the present for them and they were milking it for all they could! This taught me that it isn't your condition in life that causes distress or happiness but your attitude towards it. Enjoying the simple things right now is part of the key to happiness. I learned from these children the wisdom of getting the best out of all my moments and of concentrating on the present instead of worrying about the past and future.

Robert Louis Stevenson said it all when he wrote: "the best things are nearest; breathe in your nostrils, light in your eyes, flowers at your feet, duties at your hand, the path of God just before you. Then do not grasp at the stars but do life's plain common work as it comes, certain that daily duties and daily bread are the sweetest things in life and will make you feel good."

Chapter Two
Believe

You must have goals for the future and concentrate at times on the future but just as important is to enjoy the present and what is going on around you.

Many depressed people spend much of their time regretting their past mistakes and worrying about what is going to happen in the future. The mentally healthy person realizes that generally speaking he will never have it any better than it is right now. You may now have and always have had everything you are ever going to have. So enjoy life right now. Especially enjoy the simple things, be sure you have some big, colorful, clearly focused pictures in your mind of the things you can do right now so the present will come alive for you and make you feel good.

If you are very ambitious and concentrate an all out effort on the future and sacrifice your present satisfaction for future success, when you achieve success you may not be able to enjoy it. You may only settle for more success, partly because you have developed the habits of hard work and sacrifice and it is difficult for you to change. You have become so conditioned to the activities, strategies and use of strong will power that brought you success that you can't give up this lifestyle. You may not be able to enjoy success because your future thinking has caused you to lose touch with the here and now. Your strategies for achieving success have replaced your goal.

Chapter Two
Believe

There is nothing wrong with dreaming of success and planning to try and develop a way to make your dreams come true. However, it is unwise and mentally unhealthy to sacrifice all the joys of the present for the possible joys of ultimate achievement. Living in the present means enjoying all the things going on around you and within yourself which make you feel good and not basing your happiness on the amount of success you must have. It means making the present moment as happy and pleasant as you can. It means sometimes doing what you feel like doing instead of what you are supposed to do to achieve your financial goals.

The satisfaction of your material desires will never make you permanently happy. Because once you make a million or whatever your goal is, you will soon want another million or something else, so enjoy what you have now and pin your satisfaction on what you have, not on what you are going to get in the future. Make your goal to become a great person rather than to achieve excess material wealth. Your happiness depends on what you become, not on what you gain or achieve.

Here is a simple statement that you should say over and over to yourself whenever you get an opportunity. The ideal is to say this to yourself in a positive, convincing voice as many times as you can when awakening in the morning and before going to bed at night. Do this for one week with this commandment and then next week do it with the second commandment. In ten weeks,

Chapter Two
Believe

you have covered all the mental health commandments. Then start all over again.

"I believe in God which gives me the strength and energy to achieve my goals."

Visualize yourself with a very positive attitude in the face of adversity because of your strong beliefs and your inner strength. Turn up the brightness of this picture, in your mind. Focus it accurately, make it large and colorful. See it clearly and feel very positive. Step out of the picture and see yourself in it behaving in a very dynamic manner .

This will motivate you to believe in your strength and to know that you can take defeats and reverses as learning experiences rather than as losing experiences. It will show you how believing in yourself can carry you over adversities and you can still feel good.

Become self actualized. This means to be using all the talents you have. Some research has proven that you can't be happy unless you are doing everything you are capable of doing.

Improve your breathing. Are you breathing from your chest? To determine how you are breathing now, sit on a chair, slide forward a couple of inches, put your hands on top of one another on your

Chapter Two
Believe

stomach, as you breathe do your hands move up and down. If so you are breathing from your stomach which is good.

If your hands aren't moving you are breathing from your chest and will be taking in much less air. Try to change your breathing from your chest to your stomach so you will get the benefit of more air.

The Good Book of Godliness

Notes

The Good Book of Godliness

Notes

Chapter Three

Chant

Chanting has a spiritual impact. Great symphony orchestras, violinists and pianists touch the soul when they play delightful music. Probably the most stimulating sounds come from military parade bands, which excite you and lift you up and activate your eustress. Jazz bands are equally stimulating in a different way. Romantic music can activate the passions and excite the loving instincts of those who dance or listen.

Sound and repetition are two very powerful stimulants. Chanting has them both. By chanting aloud and repeating your chant, you can bring eustress to your body. Some one once explained the repetition of chanting by saying, "God isn't always listening. So you have to repeat."

Chanting bridges the gap between body and soul. By chanting prayers or affirmations you can rouse the spiritual feelings in yourself. It's sort of a combination of prayer and meditation.

Chapter Three
Chant

Spiritual masters chant to try and contact the divine. One saint described chanting as an ancient practise to join the worldly and the spiritual. Chanting helps to relieve distress and bring you eustress which is positive stress which comes when you succeed at something.

Sounds of chanting enter the body through the skin and bones and stimulate the nervous system. It is well known that your tone of voice communicates as much as what you say. This reveals the power of sound.

I first became aware of the beneficial effects of sounds and music when I visited a sing along bar in a small hotel. Everyone was singing with all their hearts and it made me want to sing. Each time I visited this sing along bar, I had eustress going for me. It was the sound, the repetition and the group effort.

When I started to write this piece on chanting. I felt that maybe I should skip it because I had little real experience with chanting. As I read more about it and thought about my experiences, I realized that I had been working with a form of chanting for nearly fifty years.

In my management seminars, I had a technique for loosening up my audience and relaxing them, which was a form of chanting. Here's how it worked. Often on a Monday morning, I would

Chapter Three
Chant

have forty or fifty grim looking managers who were unhappy at the thought of taking a seminar. To get them in a better mood, I would ask them to stand up, hold their arms up in a 90 degree angle in front of them and look upward. They did this reluctantly. Then I would get them to follow me and jog around the room smiling and chanting. "I am happy. I am happy. I am happy."

The results were like magic. The group now turned from a sullen quiet crowd to a joyful friendly gang. They were relaxed, laughing and talking to one another. The sound and the repetition and the moving around had really loosened them up and brought them into a happier state.

Although they resisted at first, they ended up enjoying the laughter and playfulness.

At the time I didn't realize that this was a form of chanting and I used it successfully for many years on groups of up to 200

How do you chant? Just say the words in a strong forced manner in a clipped sharp tone with plenty of expression and fairly loud. Repetition is important. The words you use will have an impact and so will the repetition and the sound. You have three elements at work.

Chapter Three
Chant

I understand that most chanters sit down. Others stand. My preference is to move around to try and get the body into the act. I like to raise my hands up in front of me to an angle of 45 degrees and look upward, smiling. Instead of standing still, I like to jog around, which helps me to stimulate eustress.

My favorite words for a chant are. "I am happy, I am happy." Another chant is to repeat the phrase, "I am healthy. I am healthy." Other good words for a chant are "I am cheerful, joyful, happy, laughing."

You can also use your name for a chant. There is something magic in your name and chanting it increases your self-esteem. Your prayers and your affirmations also make good chanting material.

To make your chanting effective, focus on your words or phrases and put your heart and voice into it. Punctuate your chant with pauses and make it punchy. You should be presenting it in a voice that sounds like singing and talking combined.

Chanting can be very helpful in activating the good feeling of eustress. Keep using your prayers and spiritual affirmations when you chant.

For example, I chant to this prayer, "Thank you God, I love you God, forgive me God, please help me God and help others. I

Chapter Three
Chant

am grateful God." I also chant this affirmation. "I am positive, optimistic, enthusiastic and in excellent physical mental and spiritual health."

The reason for chanting is to change your mood from sadness to the happiness of eustress and change your attitude from worldly thinking to spiritual thinking and eliminate distress.

Most of the great religions of the world have used chanting to help people become spiritually enlightened and connected with the Divine Presence. It is only recently that science has realized that chanting is good for physical, mental and spiritual health and will bring on eustress.

Fortunately chanting is not difficult to learn and each person can develop a technique, which fits his or her temperamental needs.

My feeling is that chanting is as important as prayer and meditation in helping a person to avoid distress. It gives us another path to God. I hope you will keep an open mind and learn to chant. It has been very helpful to me in developing spiritual fitness and activating eustress.

Notes

Chapter Four

Develop Your Self-Esteem

You can feel good immediately by realizing that you are a worthwhile person, regardless of what terrible things you think you have done. Why are you worthwhile? Just because you are you! You were created by some Super Universal Power and you have within you a spark of Unlimited Greatness.

If I go to your funeral some day, you will still be there. Your body is there and if we open your skull your brain will still be there. But obviously something is missing. What is it? The spirit which was you has gone. Let's call it the "Self."

This "self" is part of the great Universal Power. When you believe this, your state will change and you will suddenly behave like a more worthwhile person. Your "self" is perfect and that alone should make you feel good. That doesn't mean that you are perfect. Your attitudes and limited wisdom and many other things make you less than perfect. But the "self" is the perfect

Chapter Four
Develop Your Self-Esteem

part of you. It's the part of you that your friends and family like to hang out with.

Self-esteem has nothing to do with conceit, assertiveness, aggressiveness or any tendencies to self aggrandizement or showing off. These traits are all symptoms of low esteem. Self-esteem is not self-confidence: it is not attained by achievement, money, fame, or great skill. Self-esteem is just the feeling that you are worthwhile. Not because of the things you have accumulated, or the position you have achieved, or the skills you have developed but just because you are you.

How can you measure your self-esteem? Here is a rough way to appraise yourself in this regard. Just for one minute think of the person in the world you admire the most. Your father, mother, brother, sister, best friend, boss, girlfriend, boy friend, son or daughter. Now think about this person for a moment. Now think about yourself. Do you feel the same about yourself as you do about the person you admire? If so, you have good self-esteem.

People with high self-esteem are modest and unassuming. They are confident and they don't boast or social climb or drop names or practice religious or racial prejudice. They don't need to do these things to try and impress others because they know they are worthwhile the way they are.

Chapter Four
Develop Your Self-Esteem

The first step toward improving your self-esteem is to stop feeling that it is wrong to think well of yourself. Here are some statements to help you with your self esteem.

1. Stop feeling that it is wrong to like yourself

2. You are a unique and special individual. There is nobody like you and there never will be anyone like you

3. Stop criticizing yourself and putting yourself down.

4. Get more knowledge so you will behave in a wiser manner

5. Convince your subconscious mind that you are worthwhile. Affirmations will help you with this.

6. Develop yourself physically. Diet and exercise will help you. Buy clothes to improve your appearance.

7. Develop an attitude of service. What can you contribute to the world?

8. Develop greater wisdom.

9. Visualize yourself behaving like someone with high self esteem.

Chapter Four
Develop Your Self-Esteem

10. Give up boasting and telling lies about your performance.

11. Create visuals for your life line of you performing like a person with self-esteem. Keep watching these visuals.

Because most of us have been trained to be overly modest and to consider the interests of others, we sometimes feel that it is wrong to think we are worthwhile. The truth is that if you don't think well of yourself, you won't think well of others. You can have only one standard of human relations and that will apply to how you feel about yourself and about other people.

The next step toward self esteem is to realize that you are a unique and special individual. Actually, you are a spirit, a part of the great universe. As such, you are a special and worthwhile person and you should start to feel this way immediately. There is no one else exactly like you and there never will be anyone else exactly like you. The feeling that you are a part of the great universe should help you to think that you are worthwhile.

The third step is to stop criticizing yourself and putting yourself down. You are probably critical of yourself because of some of the unwise things you have done in the past. Forget it. You did the best you could with the temperament and ability you were born with and with the training you got as a child. You had no control over these things and yet they have a big influence on your behavior.

Chapter Four
Develop Your Self-Esteem

So stop blaming yourself. You are great regardless of what you have done in the past. Of course, you must take responsibility for your past behavior even though you couldn't have done it differently. If you did anything wrong, you must be punished for it.

Fortunately, you do have some control over your future. Now you can increase your self-esteem by developing more wisdom so you will behave in a wiser manner.

As your behavior improves, you will feel better about yourself. Once you get to really like yourself, you will start to feel good. You will smile and laugh more and get greater enjoyment from life. You will stop asserting yourself, demanding your rights and being aggressive. This behavior will not be necessary once you accept the fact that you are a worthwhile person. Instead, you will consider the interests of others and be ready to help them with their problems.

The fourth step is to convince your subconscious mind that you are worthwhile. This is important because probably 80% of your behavior is dictated by your subconscious. To activate your subconscious you should practice affirmations. You can do this by having a sentence or phrase which you keep repeating whenever you have any spare time. The subconscious will do what you tell it, if your directions are strong and clear, have feeling behind them, and are repeated constantly.

Chapter Four
Develop Your Self-Esteem

So here is your statement. Keep saying it over and over until it gets through to your subconscious. Then your subconscious will start to respond by directing you in how to behave to have good self-esteem:

Every day in every way I like myself more and more. I know that I am a worthwhile person and that I can be great.

You can use a variety of statements in this regard:

"I like myself: I deserve to have people love me: I am a worthwhile person just because I am me: I don't have to prove my worth: I feel good about myself: I forgive myself for any wrong I have done."

Writing down these affirmations as well as saying them aloud will help to register them on your subconscious mind and thereby improve your self-esteem.

A fifth step is to develop yourself physically. A program of exercising and eating the right foods can get you into good physical condition so you will feel proud of your body. This will help you to feel you are more worthwhile. Dressing can also help. Buy yourself the best clothes you can afford and be proud of your appearance. Always be neat and clean. Respect yourself.

Chapter Four
Develop Your Self-Esteem

For the sixth step you can change your attitudes and develop an attitude of service. Think of what you can contribute to the world, not what you can get from it. Take a positive stance in every situation. Look at what is good in yourself, in others, and in the world around you. As you practice this positive approach, you will think better of yourself. Work always to a standard of excellence so you will get satisfaction and pride from achievement.

The seventh step in your progress toward self esteem is to develop greater wisdom; this will help you to make wiser decisions, which will make you feel better about yourself. So increase your knowledge by reading and studying in many fields. Widen your interests so you will be exposed to a greater range of activities and people. Get active in group organizations and try to meet as many interesting people as possible. We learn more from other people than from any other source.

Try to meet the wisest and most intelligent people. Listen to them and find out how they think and what their attitudes are. Copy their thinking and physical behavior and you will pick up some of their confidence and self-esteem.

Visualization and self talk have great power over your subconscious mind and your behavior. You are controlled by the pictures you carry in your mind and your life line and by what you say to yourself. Your behavior is controlled by your self-image and self talk.

Chapter Four
Develop Your Self-Esteem

If you want to have better self-esteem, start visualizing yourself behaving like someone with high self-esteem and hang a picture of this on your life line in the immediate future. Keep telling yourself that you have a high regard for yourself. Be modest and consider the interests of others. Stop criticizing yourself and others.

Your life line is an imaginary vision in your mind of your entire life.

It's like a clothes line on which you have everything hanging that has ever happened to you and everything hanging that is going to happen to you

Give up boasting, telling white lies about your performance, name dropping, social climbing, and showing prejudice. These are all symptoms of lack of self-esteem. When you behave in any of these ways, take a few minutes and visualize how you would behave in these circumstances if you had high self-esteem. Eventually you will get into the habit of running your high self-esteem tapes through your mind and gradually your behavior will change to that of a person with high self-esteem.

Day-dream as much as you can about what you will be like when you have self-esteem. Visualize yourself as capable of building other people up and listening to them talk without demanding

Chapter Four
Develop Your Self-Esteem

the floor so you can tell how great you are. When you have self-esteem, you won't need to prove that you are the greatest.

See yourself accepting criticisms from others or complaints about your work without becoming upset. Hang a picture of this on your life line. You know you are a worthwhile person and therefore the rejections and put downs of others don't distress you.

Allow others to disagree with you without being overly sensitive and becoming hostile and losing control. Don't be upset if someone seems to be getting more favourable treatment than you while waiting for service in a store or restaurant. Keep control and quietly ask for better service without blaming the clerk or waiter in a hostile, childish manner. You don't have to prove that you are just as good as everyone else. You know you are a worthwhile person.

Create visuals for your life line of you performing like a person who has a high self-esteem and keep watching yourself in these high self-esteem roles. Increasing your self-esteem will help you to be more effective at your work. Unless you feel that you are worthwhile, you will fail to get promotions because you will think that you are not good enough for a higher ranking job. You will also find it difficult to establish a satisfactory relationship with another person. Who would want to love a nobody like you? This kind of thinking will make you jealous, suspicious and possessive and could kill a good relationship with your partner. It will also

Chapter Four
Develop Your Self-Esteem

be difficult for you to find real happiness if you don't feel you are a worthwhile person because you feel that you are unworthy of happiness. Whenever you feel especially good you will sabotage this feeling because you don't think you deserve it.

High self-esteem will help you in your relationships with others because if you like yourself, you will like others and they will appreciate you. On the other hand, if you hate yourself you will hate others because you can only have one standard of human behavior. Nearly all crime is committed by people who hate themselves and therefore hate others and kill and rob and rape.

Who has low self-esteem? Everybody! We are each somewhere on a scale of 1-10. If you are at 1, 2, 3 on the scale, you are probably unhappy in your personal life and not too successful in your job. If you are at 4,5, or 6 you are probably reasonably happy in your life, get along reasonably well with others and are quite successful at your job. If you are on the scale at 7, 8 or 9 you are very happy, get along very well with others and are very successful at your work. I have never yet met anyone who is a 10 on the scale but you can try for it.

How did you get low self-esteem? You start out in the world with low self-esteem. It starts in the first year of life when you are helpless and can't feed or dress or entertain yourself. Nor can you walk or talk or clean yourself. As a result, you feel useless and not very worthwhile.

Chapter Four
Develop Your Self-Esteem

If you grow up in a family with wise and understanding parents, you will be taught to think well of yourself and your self-esteem will increase. On the other hand, if you are raised by parents who push you around and keep putting you down, your feelings of low self-esteem will be accentuated. Even in normal families where the parents are loving, understanding people, they will occasionally make remarks that will affect a child's self-esteem.

When they are under pressure, overworked or worried by major problems, any parents are likely to lash out at their children call them "stupid", "sloppy" "lazy" or "useless".

These things certainly lower a child's self-esteem. Sometimes at school, children are called names like "skinny", "fatso", "fat lips", "sissy" and many other names that hurt and contribute to low self-esteem. These early put downs have a lasting impression on a person. One of my clients, whose name was Ivy, said the kids at school called her "poison ivy" and at age fifty seven she had still not quite recovered from this experience.

When you leave the family and school and go out into the real world to live, you will find the discouragements, frustrations, put downs and failures make you feel at times that you are not a worthwhile person. Keep working on your self-esteem. It won't get any better unless you consciously follow a definite program to correct it. Your self-esteem will not increase as you go through

Chapter Four
Develop Your Self-Esteem

life unless you do something to improve it. So go back over the list of remedies I have given you and keep constantly working on these methods of making you feel more worthwhile.

Is it possible to get too much self-esteem? This is a question I am often asked. The answer is a resounding "no". It would be like getting too much good health, too much understanding, too much honesty or too much positive focusing.

We all start out in life with low self-esteem. As time goes by if you convince yourself that you are worthwhile, you will be a modest, confident, unassuming person who will enjoy life and be able to get along with others and be capable of using your talents to the fullest. If you don't, you may go through life as a demanding, aggressive, prejudiced, name dropping, and social climbing person.

Confidence in yourself will certainly help you to develop self esteem. Self confidence is a feeling that you are efficient at what you are doing. It is a feeling that you are competent. Self-esteem, on the other hand, is a feeling that you are worthwhile. Self-confidence will help you to develop your self-esteem but you could be very capable at what you are doing and have a very high self-confidence and yet think that you are not a very worthwhile person. John Belushi, Janis Joplin, Elvis Presley and Marilyn Monroe were all confident in themselves but they didn't think they were worthwhile.

Chapter Four
Develop Your Self-Esteem

To develop your self-confidence, you should try to become skilful at something. Become an expert at your work, in some sport, in the arts, in the academic field, or at some type of manual or social skill. I have seen young men and women who were lacking in confidence suddenly blossom into very confident people when they became skilled at hockey, baseball, basketball, football or gymnastics. I have seen others change from shrinking violets to quite confident people when promoted to supervisory jobs which they learned to do well. Success in their work gave them confidence. When you do anything at which you can achieve, learn, create, develop skills, meet people or help people with their problems it makes you more confident. This will also improve your self-esteem and make you feel that you are a worthwhile person.

Skills in the social area are particularly good for confidence building and those who take public speaking courses often change from being self-effacing, timid people to positive, self-assured people who have confidence in themselves. Often shy, retiring people who develop an expertise as a mechanic, carpenter, counsellor, teacher, doctor, designer, dentist, engineer will gradually gain confidence in themselves. So find out the areas of your life in which you have some talent and start to develop this talent by gaining more knowledge or skills in that particular field.

Naturally, as you become more confident, you will feel that you are a more worthwhile person. However, you may have very high

Chapter Four
Develop Your Self-Esteem

self-confidence and still need to improve your self-esteem. The other techniques I have described in this chapter will help you to develop your self-esteem. Remember, self-esteem has nothing to do with being demanding, self-assertive or aggressive. These qualities indicate a person of low self-esteem. Those with high self-esteem are modest and unassuming and confident that they are worthwhile.

Self-esteem does not depend on your skills, abilities or achievements although improving yourself in any area will help you to get better self-esteem. This is not the complete answer. To have self-esteem you must believe that you are a worthwhile person just because you are you. In my book Like yourself and Live, published by Hunter Carlyle publishing, I have described in detail how you can develop your self-esteem.

Life Line Exercise

What I would like you to do is fly out in your imagination ination over your life line and fly down into a place about one month from now. Create a mental image of a scene in which you are acting with great self-esteem. Somebody has challenged something you said and instead of losing your temper and lashing out at that person you are calm, cool and collected asking that person what they mean. Get right into this picture, enjoying your high self-esteem behavior. Make

Chapter Four
Develop Your Self-Esteem

the picture brighter, larger, more clearly focused and bring it close to you. Make it move or do anything that will give it a greater impact. Wallow in it and enjoy the great feeling and the beautiful sounds and what you are seeing. Next I want you to step out of the picture and see yourself in it as you hang it on your life line. Now fly up over your life line and back to the present.

This vision will now be registered on your subconscious mind through your life line, and as you move into the future your subconscious mind will be working to help you develop the self-esteem needed to behave in the way you have acted in the picture on your life line.

So keep working on all the ideas in this chapter and keep repeating your affirmation statement whenever you have any feelings that you are useless or worthless or anytime you reveal low self-esteem in your day to day behavior. Take charge, turn things around and keep repeating this affirmation.

I like myself and I know that I
am a worthwhile person.

Gradually you will get to feel that you are worthwhile and your state will change and you will feel excited and stimulated.

The Good Book of Godliness

Notes

Chapter Five

Enjoy!

Laugh and the world laughs with you because laughing makes everyone feel good. Laugh and smile as much as you can. Whenever you are in a good state you can move yourself quickly into a better state by laughing and smiling.

How can you get yourself to laugh right now? It is easy. Just create an artificial laugh. Just chant,"Ha ha ha - ha ha ha - ha ha ha," and your state will begin to change. Keep up this artificial laugh and smile at the same time. Stand straight and look up. Keep moving around and visualize yourself being happy and joyful and you should soon improve your state. If you do it right, you can anchor joyous, happy feelings to your artificial laugh.

Think of one of the funniest incidents you can remember. Try to get the feeling of that humorous situation. Visualize yourself right back in that incident and in a great humorous state. Think of what you saw and heard and how you felt on that occasion. How

Chapter Five
Enjoy!

were you standing or sitting? Make the mental picture brighter, clearer, more colorful, larger and move it in close to yourself. Reproduce your posture and what you saw, heard and felt, now at the height of your humorous feeling take a deep breath and chant, "Ha ha ha - ha ha ha - ha ha ha," and at the same time press your thumbs against your forefingers.

Linger mentally in this humorous situation and do your artificial laugh several times pressing your thumbs and forefingers together. You should now be anchored to this joyous situation and you should be able to bring this feeling back anytime by going, "Ha ha ha - ha ha ha - ha ha ha," and pressing your thumbs and forefingers together. Try it. If it doesn't work the first time, keep trying.

You can also anchor yourself to other happy, fun situations in the same way. Go back in your imagination and get the exact feeling of fun you had in another situation. What did you see, hear and feel. How were you sitting and standing. Turn up the brightness, make it colourful, large, clearly focused and move it close to yourself. Try to reproduce it exactly as you experienced it. Now at the height of the fun when the punch line has been told, take a deep breathe and repeat "Ha ha ha - ha ha ha - ha ha ha," and press your thumbs and forefingers together on each hand. Hold this feeling for a while and repeat the exercise several times. Now you have anchored yourself to another fun situation that will make you feel good anytime you want it.

Chapter Five
Enjoy!

Have you ever been in a depressed mood and then somebody made a humorous comment or a funny joke and suddenly you broke into laughing and into a new state of mind and body? It happened immediately. Or have you every been in a solemn group where there is some conflict and it looks as if things are turning into a fighting situation and someone suddenly makes a humorous comment and in a flash everyone starts to laugh and immediately all are felling good?

Laughing and smiling are two of the fastest ways to put yourself and others into a favorable state. So I am going to explore with you some of the ways you can use laughter to change states quickly. I will also look into the possibility of using humor in your life to constantly help keep you feeling good. I put humor in this book to lighten it up so you wouldn't become too grimly serious in your pursuit of feeling good. Comedians earn fabulous incomes because they can take a group of tired, worried business men or women and can suddenly change their states and get them smiling and laughing. Bill Cosby is one of the highest paid entertainers in the world because he can make people laugh and move them up from a good state to an excellent state in a flash. Humorous books, movies and TV shows are the greatest state changers in our modern society.

People with a sense of humor who can bring fun and laughter into almost any situation are the most popular because we all want to

Chapter Five
Enjoy!

feel good and we welcome anyone who can help us do it. Men who have the most success with women are those who can make them laugh. When a woman starts to laugh she changes state, feels good and looks favorably on the man who can do it. In the human relations area, laughter is one of the best techniques for getting along with people of both sexes and gaining their support. A woman with a sense of humor is desirable to a man because when she gets him laughing, she puts him in a state to feel good.

In the public speaking business, the best communicators are those who lard their serious comments with funny lines. People like to laugh because it makes them feel good. They like to be entertained while they are learning. The highest paid speakers are humorists as well as educators.

How much do you laugh? How much do you smile?Are you enjoying life? How much pleasure are you getting out of life? These are the first questions I would ask you to determine your mental health. If you laugh and snile all the time you will feel good.

How much you laugh will tell if all is well. It will tell me if you are enjoying life and feeling good and are in a good state. These are the clues that indicate you are free of distress and depression. If you are unhappy and worried about something and are not feeling good, I can immediately put you in a good state if I can get you laughing or smiling.

Chapter Five
Enjoy!

Because the main symptom of mental ill health is unhappiness, worry and depression, it seems to me the front line of attack against mental ill health should be to try and keep happy. Let's put it this way: when you start to over worry and get depressed, this is a signal that something is wrong. You are either doing something that is unhealthy or you are thinking in a way that prevents you from feeling good.

You can do much to bring more fun and humor into your life by anchoring yourself to humorous situations and by using your "Ha ha ha - ha ha ha - ha ha ha," and thumbs pressing on forefingers to recall these humorous states. You can also bring more humor into your life by visualizing yourself as a humorous person. Another way to become more humorous is to get your subconscious mind slanted in a humorous direction.

The first step towards seeing the humorous side of things and enjoying life is to understand that with all the different types of people in the world and the many different situations we have to face, there are bound to be some unusual things happen. Don't expect too much too soon from life and you won't be disappointed when things don't work out exactly as you planned. Don't take yourself and life too seriously. It's a game. Play it as well as you can, but don't expect to be perfect or even near perfect. You win some and you lose some as you go through life.

Chapter Five
Enjoy!

Nothing is more important than laughter in your growth and development. When you are laughing, it is natures signal that you are feeling good, making progress and enjoying life. Experiencing pleasure is a very positive feeling. It gives you strength to do all the things you must do for success. It makes you more confident and helps you to think well of yourself. It enables you to appreciate life and all its blessings. It keeps you in a good state. Humor is only found in an imperfect world. Laughter and humor are ways of dealing with the world's shortcomings.

I urge you to get pleasure from doing things and achieving, learning, creating, developing your skills, traveling, meeting new people, or helping people with their problems. Doing these things will make you feel good. Relaxing, meditating, philosophizing and day-dreaming can also make you feel good. These inner pleasures can be just as great as the pleasures that come from activities.

Unfortunately, many people are unable to enjoy fully the joys of living. They may have been trained to reject pleasure and have been taught to take responsibility too seriously, to keep their noses to the grindstone and work hard. They may not have been taught that fun and laughter and pleasure can sometimes save their lives by relieving stress and helping them to roll with the punches, and feel good in the present.

Chapter Five
Enjoy!

Many people who are striving to be rich and famous are unhappy because they are always looking forward to the day when they will have more money or be prime minister or president. There is nothing wrong with being ambitious, but there are many things wrong with passing up present joy and pleasure for an uncertain future.

In our day-to-day struggle to survive and make a living, we have all become too serious. The grim pursuit of work and the difficulties of getting the job done have absorbed us so much that we have put laughter, pleasure, having fun and enjoying life on the back burner. The pursuit of achievement, power, money and status has taken over and we are in a more serious state than nature intended.

The original man in the jungle was a playful, fun loving person who had to struggle to eat and survive but his capacity to play and laugh and enjoy life and keep in a relaxed state gave him relief from stress, fear and insecurity. He didn't return home to his cave with ulcers because other cavemen had collected more bananas than he. Playing and laughing were a very important part of life in the jungle. Animals know how to play and relax by gamboling and stretching and dozing in the sun. They get pure pleasure from their present environment, which makes them feel good. They don't worry or fret about past events or have heated arguments with their stockbrokers.

Chapter Five
Enjoy!

Mentally healthy people are in a happy state. Mentally sick people are generally in an unhappy and depressed state. So if you want to keep mentally healthy, get some fun into your life. Relax and play more and enjoy life and laugh and smile as much as possible. This will make you feel good. If you can do this you will get along better with people and be more effective at your work.

Action always comes first. If you want to be confident, act confident and you will eventually be confident. If you want to be happy, act happy. If you want to enjoy life, act as if you are enjoying it. So sing, whistle,laugh and smile whenever you can. Act happy and you will be happy. Keep using your artificial laugh, "ha ha ha - ha ha ha - ha ha ha," and press your thumbs and forefingers together.

There is much evidence that fun and humor contribute to physical health. Throughout history, the great thinkers and philosophers have been telling us that humor and laughter are therapeutic. Freud said that humor was a good way to counteract nervous tension. Emmanuel Kant said that laughter produces a feeling of good health and stimulates the body processes.

Probably our best example of how effective laughter can be in the health area comes from Norman Cousins, author of Anatomy of an Illness (Bantam books). In his book, he describes how he

Chapter Five
Enjoy!

helped cure himself of an apparently incurable physical disease by thinking positively and laughing as much as possible.

Norman Cousins had been advised by his doctors that he had a crippling disease they believed was incurable and that his chances of survival were very slight. He decided to abandon traditional medical treatment and to treat himself by trying to stimulate his positive feelings to see if he couldn't improve his body chemistry. He decided to try and think positively and laugh as much as possible.

He arranged to get amusing movies such as reruns of the old television show "Candid Camera" and some old Marx Brothers' movies. He soon found that ten minutes of laughter had a positive effect on his physical condition. He kept watching humorous films and also had his nurses read him humorous books to try and keep him laughing.

The treatment worked and Norman Cousins started to get better. He proved scientifically that his laughing treatment was working by taking blood sedimentation readings before and after each session of laughing. Each time he did this there was a drop of about five points. This trend stayed with him and gave him a gradual improvement. He was excited to learn that there was a physiological basis for the theory that laughter is good for you.

Chapter Five
Enjoy!

Norman Cousins was learning of the tremendous capacity of the human mind and body to recover, even under adverse conditions, and that there is a natural drive in the human mind and body toward good health. Appreciating and protecting this drive is equally important to us all. The way to do it is to keep enjoying life, keep laughing as much as possible and get plenty of exercise.

Unfortunately, humor which triggers laughter is very difficult to generate. We continue to tell the same old jokes with variations, and comedians steal jokes and funny situations from one another, because to produce humor is a very difficult task. Will Rogers, Stephen Leacock, Woody Allen, James Thurber, Mark Twain, Dorothy Parker, Groucho Marx and a few other writers and performers have been able to create original humor and we revere them for this rare talent. Bob Hope, George Burns, Bill Cosby, Eddie Murphy, Red Skelton, Johnny Carson and many other comedians have become rich because our society is willing to pay a big price in order to laugh.

Let me alert you to some of the benefits that can come to you from laughing. Physiologically, laughing stimulates your blood circulation and exercises your lungs. It also exercises your diaphragm, which is a muscle between your chest and your stomach. If you put your hand on your stomach while you are

Chapter Five
Enjoy!

laughing, you will feel your diaphragm moving up and down, exercising the muscles in this area of your body.

When you laugh, it causes you to breathe more deeply and take more oxygen into your body. The entire heart-lung-blood delivery system benefits when you laugh. Laughter is very relaxing to your body as well as to your mind and emotions. When you laugh at something, you forget your problems, at least temporarily.

The experts tell us that laughter produces endorphins in the brain which reduce pain. When you laugh at something you get a new slant on life because you become less intense, more objective and not so deeply involved. The desire to feel good and be happy is the greatest need of human beings.

Some great thinkers have said that the purpose of life is to feel good. Feeling good is an indication that your life is going well and you are in a good state. Having pleasure and enjoying life, laughing and smiling may be the secrets of success. This is why successful people tend to be fun-loving people. When I first discovered this, I thought that these people were happy because they were successful. But I later found that they were successful because they were happy.

Laughing and having fun stimulates the pituitary gland, which has an influence on your energy and vitality, so necessary to

Chapter Five
Enjoy!

success. Enjoyment and pleasure will stimulate you and put you in a relaxed state. So laugh as much as possible. Search out things that bring you pleasure and be as active as possible in these things. Start to enjoy yourself right now. Begin with the simple pleasures of reading, visiting with friends, walking in the country and enjoying the beauty of nature.

Why is laughing so important to you and so therapeutic? It's because many things happen physically and psychologically when you laugh.

The following excerpt will indicate the extent to which laughter activates the body physically.Richard Boston, in his book An Anatomy of Laughers (Collins, London 1974) gives the fullest description of laughter he has come across, taken from GVN Dearborn (Science 1st, June 1900):

"There occurs in laughter and more or less in smiling, chronic spasms of the diaphragm in number ordinarily about eighteen perhaps and contraction of most of the muscles of the face. The upper side of the mouth and its corners are drawn upward. The upper eyelid is elevated as are also, to some extent, the brows, the skin over the glabella, and the upper lip, while the skin at the outer canthi of the eyes

Chapter Five
Enjoy!

is characteristically puckered. The nostrils are moderately dilated and drawn upward, the tongue slightly extended, the cheeks distended and drawn somewhat upward; in persons with the pinnal muscles largely developed, the pinnal tend to incline forwards. The lower jaw vibrates or is somewhat withdrawn (doubtless to afford all the possible air to the distended lungs) and the head, in extreme laughter, is thrown backward; the truck is straightened even to the beginning of bending backward; until (and this usually happens soon) fatigue-pain in the diaphragm and accessory muscles causes a marked proper flexion of the trunk for its relief. The whole arterial vascular system is dilated, with consequent blushing from the effect of the capillaries of the back and neck, and at times the scalp and the hands. From this same cause in the main the eyes often slightly bulge forwards and the lachrymal gland becomes active, ordinarily to a degree only to cause a "brightening" of the eyes, but often to such an extent that the tears overflow entirely their proper channels."

Chapter Five
Enjoy!

Some writers have declared laughter to be beneficial because it restores homeostasis, stabilizing blood pressure, oxygenating the blood, massaging the vital organs, stimulating circulation, facilitating digestion, relaxing the system and making you feel good.

In spite of these physical changes that take place when you laugh. I am sure that the psychological and emotional changes are even more important. The playful attitude that encompasses you and the resulting relaxation are the most therapeutic actions you could take for relieving stress. You can't be suffering from distress when you are laughing. Try to worry and laugh at the same time. It's impossible.

To me this means that we should take action in our lives which will bring us pleasure and cause us to feel good. If successful mentally healthy people are happy people who enjoy fun and laughing one of the best routes to success and happiness is to search for all the things in your life that you like to do, that you do well and that make you feel good and give you pleasure. Spend as much time doing these things as you can so you will enjoy life and laugh as much as possible.

Laughter is something spontaneous that comes upon us when we see or hear something that we think is funny. Psychologists have tried to discover what makes us laugh. Their findings indicate that it is something that changes our train of thought suddenly. If

Chapter Five
Enjoy!

your mind is following a certain line of reasoning and suddenly it is changed, then the surprise of the change will make you laugh.

I experimented with my granddaughter when she was two years old. In playing peek-a-boo with her, she looked quite puzzled as I struck my head around a wall and said "Peek-a-boo". If I got down on my knees and peeked at her from a completely different position, she smiled and broke out laughing. Each time I fooled her, and appeared in an unexpected place, it was funny.

Humor can also come from exaggeration. For example, I heard a mature speaker say that he had no enemies. He had outlived them all. This was an exaggeration, of course, but funny because it was unexpected. The same could be achieved with an understatement. Groucho Marx at one time was considering suing a certain publication for slandering him. His lawyers were planning to take the case to court but Groucho said first he would write to the publishers and see if he could get them to be reasonable. So he wrote that unless they published a retraction for the article about him he would cancel his subscription to their magazine. This was an unexpected reply and understatement. The unexpected can also come about by suddenly changing a train of thought. For example "You can keep young by dieting and exercising, and by lying about your age." This last comment is funny because it changes a train of thought.

Chapter Five
Enjoy!

Another way to get a laugh is with the humorous catalogue. This is a situation where you have a list of items to which you add an item at the end of the list that is unexpected and out of context. For example, I might say that he is a great golfer because he has a smooth swing, putts accurately, chips and pitches with precision and he can't add. The last item is out of context and unexpected and will get a smile or a snicker or a belly laugh depending on to whom you are telling it.

So keep watching for situations where you can exaggerate, understate, suddenly change the train of thought or create a humorous catalogue and you should be able to create some humor as you go your daily rounds. Of course, there are other ways but these are the best. Create humor to amuse yourself and get into the habit of seeing the fun in life. Don't expect many brilliantly funny lines. Creating humor is very difficult. If you can do it easily and effortlessly, you will be able to make many millions a year like Bill Cosby.

When you awaken each morning, if you have trouble swinging into action, sit on the side of your bed and reproduce your artificial laugh in order to get your day started right. Go "ha ha ha - ha ha ha - ha ha ha," and press your thumbs and forefingers together. This will do several things for you. First it will start some of the positive physical and psychological activities in your body that are triggered by laughing and make you feel good.

Chapter Five
Enjoy!

It will also alert you to the fact that you shouldn't take life or yourself too seriously and that you should have all the fun you can. It will bring back those joyful feelings that are anchored to your artificial laugh.

The emphasis throughout this book is on enjoying life and having all the pleasure and fun you can while pursuing your goals and contributing to the world as much as possible. The theory is that by having fun, laughing and smiling and you will experience the positive feelings of a good mental state. It is when you are unhappy and in a distressed state that I will start to worry about your mental health.

To change yourself to a fun-loving person, your life line can be very helpful. Let's put an image of you being a fun-loving, happy person on your life line which is a line in your mind which represents your life history. It's like a clothes line with all the things that have happened and are going to happen in your life hanging on it.

Life Line Exercise

Visualize yourself in a scene where you are laughing and joking with some of your friends. Get right into this picture. What do you hear, what do you feel, and what do you see? Turn up the brightness on this picture, make it larger, clearly focused and

Chapter Five
Enjoy!

more colourful. Move it in closer. Now take a step out of this scene and be disassociated. See yourself in the picture laughing and having fun with your friends as you hang it on your life line. This will motivate your subconscious mind into making you a fun loving, happy person. Whenever you are looking over your life line in the future and adjusting it, you will see this picture of you in a cheerful state enjoying life. This will renew your thrust in the direction of being a more relaxed, fun loving person.

Here is your affirmation statement for laughing. Keep repeating it constantly as you visualize yourself laughing and enjoying life.

I am smiling and laughing, having fun
and pleasure and feeling good.

The Good Book of Godliness
Notes

The Good Book of Godliness
Notes

Chapter Six

Future!

Be in charge, take command, and control your destiny. Feel powerful and ecstatic with the joy of knowing you are the captain of your life and know exactly where you are going and how you are going to get there.

It all depends on your state and you can change your state immediately by imagining yourself flying up over your life line. See your whole life spread out beneath you from birth to age 110. This will give you a sense of power and control over your life and should immediately change your state. One hundred and ten years may seem like a long time but Moses lived to 300 and Methuselah to 800, so why not you to 110?

It's exciting to be presiding over your entire life knowing that you can drift down into your life line and change anything you want. You can go back in your past, reenact events and change your impression of them. You can go into the future and plan

Chapter Six
Future!

things for your future as you want them to happen. They may not happen exactly as you planned but close to how you planned them. What a sense of power and control. Yes you can motivate yourself and change your attitudes and control the direction of your life.

In order to be in charge, you must first set an outcome. Without a specific goal to aim at, you will drift aimlessly, controlled by the whims of circumstance and led down one garden path after another, ending up confused and blaming the system for your failure to achieve the things you are capable of achieving. Find out exactly what you want from life and communicate it loudly and clearly to your subconscious mind by hanging it on your life line. Don't forget that your subconscious mind is responsible for 80% of what you do. So get it working for you and you will be a winner.

I know the outcome you would like to have. You want to feel good or be in a good state. Why do I know this? Because everybody wants to feel good. This is the goal of every living person. We all want to feel good but each of us has a different way of getting those good feelings. What will put you in a feeling good state will be different than what will put me in this state? So it's important that you discover the key to making yourself feel good.

The guidelines to getting the outcome you want are as follows:

Chapter Six
Future!

1. Your goals should conform to your values. Do you want to make piles of money or do you want to dedicate your life to helping others? Is independence the most important thing to you or are you more concerned with thinking, being creative or becoming more efficient? Until you truly establish what you value most, you won't really be happy. There is no point in achieving a goal that you don't really want. Here again is the list of values on which you can rate yourself. Use these values to set your outcome. Pick out the things that you value most and create a career based on these things. Let your imagination run wild. If you can imagine it, you can probably do it.

1. Money or material things	13. Health
2. Security	14. Thinking and philosophizing
3. Efficiency	15. Peace of mind
4. Helping others	16. Power
5. Health	17. Honesty
6. Self-esteem	18. Loyalty
7. The esteem of others	19. Team work
8. Creativity	20. Love
9. Freedom and independence	21. Family
10. Sociability	23. Companionship
11. Success	24. Peace of Mind
12. Opportunity	25. Physical Activity

2. When you have decided on the values that are important to you, try to spell out why you want these goals. Sure, they will

Chapter Six
Future!

make you feel good. But why will they make you feel good? If you choose money as one of your values, why do you want it? Because you will be able to travel, live in a big home, buy a yacht, join a country club, give money to charity, start a business? Spell out in detail why you want the money.

Maybe you want to study philosophy or write a book or solve complex mathematical problems or get a university degree. Spell it out.

Why you do something is more important than how you do it. If you sort out your most important values and make sure your outcome satisfies these values, then think of all the reasons you want to achieve these goals, then you will be motivated to achieve them. Your values will give you some reasons but there may be other reasons. Think. Victor Frankl spelled it out clearly when he said, "If you have a why to live for, you can live with any how."

To stimulate yourself to think of your goals and why you want them, you could ask yourself these questions. What am I proud of? What excites me? What makes me happy? What am I grateful for? What am I hoping for?

3. Be sure to take responsibility for your life as it is. Don't blame your limitations and failures on others. You are responsible for what you are now and you can move from there to change

Chapter Six
Future!

things. If you aren't responsible, you won't be able to have what you want because your future will depend on luck and good breaks instead of on you.

4. Your goals must be positive, not negative. A goal to avoid something or stop doing something won't work. Your desired outcome must be to improve yourself or to do something or gain something.

5. Write your goals down on paper before you hang them on your life line so you can refer to them and change them when necessary. Writing them down will also reinforce your goals and rivet them into your mind.

6. Hang your goals on your life line. Fly out into the future at the point where you want to achieve each goal. Fly down into your life line and hang your goals in the right places.

7. Visualize yourself achieving your goals. See the people involved, hear what they are saying and reproduce how you will feel. Make the picture bright, large, clearly focused and colorful. Now step out of this picture and disassociate from it, watching yourself in the picture achieving your desired outcome by hanging your goals on your life line.

Chapter Six
Future!

When I am asked to make a motivational speech to a group of managers, I don't ask them to work hard. I urge them to fly out into the future on their life lines and become as creative as possible about what they want to achieve. I tell them to visualize exactly what they want as accurately and in as much detail as possible and talk to themselves in strong, positive terms.

I tell them to let themselves go, create the most beautiful pictures in their minds about what they want and describe the results they want clearly and positively. I tell them to make the pictures brighter, more colorful, larger and more focused. I urge them to concentrate on what they are hearing, seeing and feeling. Then I urge them to step out of their pictures and hang them on their life lines while they are watching themselves in the pictures.

They don't have to use will power or drive themselves to work hard, they just have to get excited about what they wish to achieve, fly out into the future at the point where they want to achieve it and create a great mental picture of them getting exactly what they want and hang it on their life lines.

As they move towards their desired outcomes, they can motivate themselves by making the pictures larger, more focused and more colorful. If they are under pressure and feel they are overworking, all they have to do is move the pictures out further on their life line and give themselves more time to achieve their goals. I show

Chapter Six
Future!

them that they can now motivate themselves and control their lives by adjusting the pictures on their life lines. They can move the pictures out into the future or in close to them. They can change the size of the pictures and make them brighter or dimmer and these changes will affect their behavior.

Giving yourself a general goal is not satisfactory because it doesn't give your mind a clear message. For example, if you tell me your goal is to become rich, I will ask you, "How rich? What do you want to see?" You may say you want fine clothes, a beautiful home, a luxurious car. Then I will ask you, "What do you want to hear?" you may say conversation with intelligent people, compliments, praise. Then I will ask you, "How do you want to feel?" your answer may be, "I want to feel important, that I count for something, that I am a somebody." What do you want to taste? "Delicious food, fine wines and champagne." What do you want to smell? "Fresh linens and perfumes and beautiful flowers."

One client of mine said his goal was to make a million dollars but when he started to measure how he would know when he achieved his goal in terms of what he would see, hear and feel, he found that he already had most of it. He was semi-retired and wanted the million to travel more so he would meet and listen to interesting people and see beautiful sights and feel good. He also wanted to buy finer clothes and a better car. I pointed out to him that he could have those things right now.

Chapter Six
Future!

He was a fairly wealthy person and could travel more and buy better things for himself but he was inclined to be overly security minded and lacked the ability to spend his money. If he had a million dollars, it wouldn't help him to achieve his goals of what he wanted to see, hear and feel. His problem was to learn how to spend wisely what he already had. He had already achieved his goal but he didn't realize it because he lacked a way to measure his goal. So maybe you have already achieved your goal but you don't know it.

To clarify what you want, I will ask you what you are seeing and hearing and feeling and smelling and tasting in your present job. Maybe you have all the things you want now. "No", you might say. "I see ordinary clothes, an average dwelling. I hear mundane conversation from dull people and I feel frustrated because I am not using my potential. I feel unappreciated and unimportant. I smell stale, decaying school rooms and I taste ordinary foods and wines and I hear young children talking constantly. I am teaching school and I feel I am capable of working with adults and teaching adults rather than children. I am a public school English teacher."

I say, "That's a very important job you have but it sounds as if you would like to make more money and improve your economic level. How would you like to teach writing skills and verbal communication skills to executives?" "Oh, I would like

Chapter Six
Future!

that. Would I have a chance of getting rich?" "Well, you could certainly make more money than at teaching school. Would you be satisfied if you could double your income? I think it would be possible to get you giving seminars for executives on "How to Speak and Write Better English". There is certainly a need for it, and you could at least double your present income by doing this."

Let's put this forward on your life line. How soon would you like to do this? "Oh, I'd like to start right now." Well, let's give you a little time to think and plan. Let's put it forward about one year in your life line. So imagine yourself flying up over your life line and seeing your entire life stretched below you from birth to 110. Now drift forward into the future to a point one year from now and visualize yourself lecturing to executives. See them in your audience, hear them talking and be aware of how elegant you feel. Make this picture brighter, more colorful, and more clearly focused. Now step out of this picture and view yourself in the picture and hang the picture on your life line. Now fly back to the present in your imagination. Your subconscious mind will now take charge and show you how to do this.

In one year you will be giving lectures to executives on "How to Speak and Write Better English". You will be hearing intelligent conversation. You will be seeing elegant people and you will feel important. This should meet all your desires for success.

Chapter Six
Future!

"Does having this take anything away from what you have now?" "Oh, I will miss some of my friends and associates but I will soon make new friends." "That's true but you will be moving around more and traveling some so you won't have the permanent connections that you have now." "I can live with that." "Will this change harm anyone in your family or among your friends?"

"Not really." "Ok. Let's go then." Always check to make sure that achieving your goal isn't going to harm anyone and that it isn't going to harm you.

What a glorious state. You're in flying up over your life line. What a feeling of power. Don't you feel now that you could be great? Don't you almost feel like Wonder woman?

Goals activate your internal drive to succeed. They give you a purpose and a reason to achieve something.

Aiming for a desired outcome gives an excitement to your activities. Setting goals will stimulate your creativity and help you come up with new ideas on how to achieve the results you want. Once you have established an outcome, your mind will show you short cuts to get there. You will manage your time better and stop wasting effort on things that don't bring you to your goal. Without goals you tend to collapse, become bored and depressed. By hanging your outcome on your life line you

Chapter Six
Future!

are adding power and the drive of your subconscious mind to the achievement of your outcome. This makes an impact on your brain so that what you want in the future will become real.

What are your limitations? Identify any weaknesses you may have and visualize yourself overcoming these weaknesses. Keep working at the pictures in your mind. Every spare minute you get, concentrate on visualizing yourself overcoming your limitations and becoming the person you want to be.

Carry this one step further by visualizing an ideal day in your life when you become successful. Construct in your mind the lifestyle and environment in which you will live. What will you see, hear, feel, taste and smell? Fly forward above your life line and create a picture of a typical day in your life. Get right into the picture and enjoy what you are hearing, seeing and feeling. Make the picture brighter, more colorful, clearly focused and larger. Then step out of the picture and hang it on your life line at whatever point in time you want to achieve it.

Don't forget that your subconscious mind has the power to give you close to what you want if you have the talent, but your mind needs an accurate description and vision of what you want. It needs to get colorful, big, clearly focused pictures hung on your life line of what you want. Supplement your visuals with positive, confident verbal comments and stronger feelings. Don't be afraid

Chapter Six
Future!

to talk to your subconscious with clear, concise directions of what you want.

The Good Book of Godliness

Notes

The Good Book of Godliness
Notes

Chapter Seven

Goals

Goals are very important. If you have goals you have something to help measure yourself with. They can be as simple as "today I am going to drink 8 glasses of water for my health" or they could be more long term and complicated like "I am going to lose 10 pounds over 6 months"

Each time you set a goal, make sure you have not set one so high that you set yourself up for failure. Commit to each goal by writing it down. Post it on your fridge so you can see it each day. Calling on God to help you with your goals is also a way to support yourself emotionally.

Other types of goals you could have is to help others. I have covered this off earlier in my book but would like to take some time to expand on it. Giving back to the community, whether it is through your community centre or to a neighbor it is a great

Chapter Seven
Goals

feeling of satisfaction. Helping organizations such as Cancer, Heart and Stroke are also good goals to set for yourself.

Each season there is a focus on different non for profit organizations, this could be a goal where you help each organization seasonally, not isolating yourself to one. As a fringe benefit you will meet new people and find new interests because of your kindness.

Many other types of goals can be set... the important thing is that you write them down. A friend of mine writes them down in the back of his calendar and visits them every day. Once he has achieved his goal he check's it off.

Sometimes he adds another, but depending on how he feels, he might just work through the list until the end and start a new list.

The Good Book of Godliness

Notes

The Good Book of Godliness

Notes

Chapter Eight

Help Others

You'll change your state immediately if you make a personal contact with somebody. Be friendly with anyone you meet, or help someone in trouble. If you find areas of agreement and situations in which you express mutual sympathy, you will start feeling good.

A close and intimate relationship with someone of the opposite sex is undoubtedly the greatest state changer available to both men and women. Physical contact with the opposite sex is exciting and will put anyone in a super state. This is why so many people are seeking a satisfactory relationship. All kinds of physical contact, from holding hands to hugging to kissing, with someone of the opposite sex, can make you feel good.

The ultimate of course is a sexual relationship and the highest state of all is the orgasm, which will make anybody feel good. This is why men and women will take the time and spend the

Chapter Eight
Help Others

money to woo someone of the opposite sex. They know there is no better way to get into a super state than to have a physical, mental and emotional relationship. So try to meet people. Join a club, take up a sport, take a course, and try and meet someone to whom you can relate.

Sometimes a feeling of love for someone of the opposite sex is so powerful that it can demobilize a person; on the other hand it can sometimes move a person to unbelievable heights. Love has moved men and women to build castles, paint pictures, write poems, create music and to do their greatest performances because they were in an exceptional loving state. Other men and women have turned to drugs, alcohol and suicide because of frustrated love.

The key to good relations with others is to like and respect them. If you like people they will respond favorably to you. If you dislike them, they will resist you. It is important that you like yourself because if you don't like yourself you won't like others. You can have only one basic attitude towards human behavior. Whatever your attitude is towards yourself, you will apply to others. If you hate yourself, you will hate others. If you like yourself, you will like others.

If you can remember that people tend to like people that are like themselves, you will have a head start in gaining their cooperation. It's quite obvious in observing human behavior that

Chapter Eight
Help Others

we turn away from people who are not like us in appearance, thought and action. The hippy dresser with blue jeans, running shoes and dirty sweatshirt is turned off by the well dressed person in a tie and neatly pressed suit. If people are different than we are, we tend to turn against them. We say we have 'differences' with people when we can't get along.

People have violent arguments over politics, religion, and economics simply because they differ in their views and their beliefs. So if you want to get along with a particular person or a group, try to be like them. You can enter another person's world and gain his or her confidence by being as much like him or her as possible. The experts in neurolinguistic programming tell us that if we stand like the other person, copy his gestures and tone of voice, we can gain his goodwill. In addition, if you agree with the person's ideas and philosophy, you should establish powerful rapport. In other words, if you can be like the other person in body and mind, you are more likely to get along with him or her.

The reason this happens is that you are getting through to his subconscious mind. The way to do this is to be like him and he will accept you and like you. We tend to like people who are like ourselves. If you want me to like you, be like me in every way possible. So pace me physically, verbally and mentally as much as you can and I will soon begin to feel that you are like me and I will like you. The result will be rapport. According to NLP

Chapter Eight
Help Others

experts, our body language and tone of voice account for much of our communication with others. Our verbal communications count for less.

This doesn't mean that you should agree with someone on something which you are against. But instead of showing your direct disagreement, you can avoid conflicts by saying, "That's an interesting viewpoint." Or "I'm glad you brought that up." Or "I see what you mean." And question her about her beliefs. This will avoid a head-on collision. The more we are like someone and the more we can agree with her, the better we can get along.

For example, if you meet someone and she says "Isn't this a great day?" you won't gain much goodwill by saying,"No, it isn't, it's a terrible day." A disagreement of any kind puts us on the wrong wave length. Supposing someone says she thinks the Blue Jays will win the World Series and you disagree. You can say, "I disagree" and introduce a discordant note or you might say, "So you're a Blue Jay fan. Why do you think they will win?" you can thus get the other person talking and draw her out without disagreeing.

In this regard it is good human relations to eliminate the words, "but" and "however." When we disagree with others, there is a tendency to apparently agree and then say, "But." For example, you might say to someone who has disagreed with you, "That's an interesting situation but have you ever thought of this?" instead

Chapter Eight
Help Others

you could say, "That's an interesting suggestion. Why do you think that is true?" or instead of saying, "I'm glad you brought that up, however I don't think it will work for this reason." You could say, "I'm glad you brought that up. What makes you think that is the right approach?" the words "but" and "however" have negative connotations so why not eliminate them when relating to others?

It is important to remember to always consider the other person's point of view. Make sure he gets what he wants from anything you are persuading him to do. If you achieve your goals at someone else's expense, you will be the loser. The person whom you have manipulated will come back to sabotage you later. So get the habit of making sure the person you are persuading or negotiating with can achieve his goals while you are achieving yours. This is called motivation.

Rotary International has a four way test that is the Rotary formula for all human relations situations.

1. Is it the truth?

2. Is it fair to all concerned?

3. Will it build goodwill and better friendships?

4. Is it beneficial to all concerned?

Chapter Eight
Help Others

Apply this test to all your human relations problems and you will gain the goodwill of those with whom you do business.

If you can remember that every person has a strong drive to feel important and gain recognition, you will approach people with the purpose of building them up rather than putting them down. By listening to her, asking her opinions and asking her advice where possible, you will demonstrate to her that you like her and respect her opinions. She will respond favorably to you when you demonstrate in your behavior and attitudes that you like her and feel that she is important.

Being tactful, diplomatic and courteous will help you make others feel respected. This doesn't mean that you have to become a fawning, agreeable to anything, people pleasing type of person. You can still be an independent thinker and stand up for what you believe, while you have respect for other people's opinions and show an interest in their ideas.

Because of different inherited temperaments, early family backgrounds and experiences, everyone sees the world in a somewhat different way. Respect the opinions of others and try to learn from them and you will gain their confidence. If you go around with the idea that other people are just cluttering up the world and have little wisdom and knowledge, you won't gain much cooperation.

Chapter Eight
Help Others

Gaining the cooperation of others will enable you to move through life avoiding friction. Helping people with their problems is a stimulating activity, and mentally healthy people are usually active in social service work of some kind. They enjoy contributing their knowledge, experience and skill to help other people. Often if you have a problem yourself, it will disappear or fade into insignificance when you start to help others who have bigger problems than you.

Your relationships with others are very important to keep you feeling good. If you have a happy family life with sympathetic understanding people in your home, this environment will instantly move you to a better state. An intimate relationship with someone who will listen to your problems and offer wise counsel and guidance can be one of the greatest assists to keeping you feeling good.

Genie Z. Laborde, in her book Fine tune Your Brain (Syntony Publishing, Palo Alt, California), suggests a way of attaining a meeting of the minds between two people who are having differences, so they can both win.

Suppose you have two partners working together in a small organization. One of the partners is doing some social service work and he wants to allow a part-time secretary of the social service organization to use his office three afternoons a week.

Chapter Eight
Help Others

The other partner objects to this because it will bring noise and confusion into a quiet, peaceful office. To try and solve this problem have each person involved in the discussion describe their outcome in terms of what they want to see, hear and feel.

Partner #1: Outcome in Sensory Terms

See: Wants to see the part-time secretary coming into the office three afternoons per week.

Hear: Wants to hear the secretary talking on the phone helping underprivileged people:

Feel: Will feel good because he is contributing something to underprivileged people.

Partner #2: Outcome in Sensory Terms

See: Neat office. Tidy, no mess.

Hear: Nothing.Peace and quiet.

Feel: Secure in having control of the office with no one to interfere with efficiency

Chapter Eight
Help Others

Partner #1: Desired Outcome

To have the part-time secretary be able to use his office facilities when he is not there.

Partner #2: Desired Outcome

To not have anyone interfering with the peace and quiet of his office when he is trying to concentrate.

The outcome: A Win-Win Situation
(worked out by negotiation between the partners)

The secretary can do her wok in the evening as well as in the afternoon. This was satisfactory to both partners so they both achieved their desired outcome and they ended up with a win-win situation. So the secretary agreed to come in each day from 5 – 8 pm.

Sometimes when each person describes in sensory terms what he wants to achieve, a solution can be reached that will satisfy both persons and a win-win situation can be reached fairly quickly.

Even though you may get along with people and be well liked, you may not be effective in influencing others. Life is one long struggle to influence people. A child is frustrated if he can't persuade

Chapter Eight
Help Others

his parents to allow him to participate in certain activities. At school he must persuade teachers and in sports he must persuade coaches and managers of teams to give him a chance. In his teens, he must persuade a girl to have a date with him and soon he must persuade someone to marry him. For a career, he must persuade someone to give him a job, and then he must persuade his boss to give him a raise and promotion.

Day to day living requires you to persuade waiters, plumbers, accountants, doctors, garage mechanics and repair men to do all the things you want done. People in a good state are most likely to persuade others to follow them and believe in them. Skill in influencing people makes life much easier, reduces stress and contributes to your ability to feel good.

Even in such careers as acting, singing and dancing, persuasion is important. Many can act and sing and dance, but only a few can persuade directors and producers to put them in a stage show, TV or movie. Many writers can produce a book but few can persuade a publisher to publish it. Anyone can run for public office but only the most persuasive can become elected, and it takes persuasive skills at the highest level to be elected prime minister or president.

In business, persuasion is the key to success. Anyone can manufacture a product but few can sell it. Most businesses that

Chapter Eight
Help Others

fail go out of business because they can't sell enough of their product at a profit to keep operating. Even in the field of medicine our greatest doctors are those with a bedside manner who can influence their patients to have confidence.

The challenge of influencing others is one of the most exciting and stimulating activities that you can undertake. It requires creativity and is very rewarding and is really what makes the world go around.

All the books on human relations claim that there is no use trying to push people to do what you want them to do. It doesn't work. When you push people, you get resistance. When you take a too direct approach and use pressure or force, you won't get people to agree with you and you will likely get them working against you. This can cause distress and tension and could prevent you from feeling good.

When you attempt to convince a person of anything, the only way you are really going to get that person to cooperate is to get him to want to cooperate. How do you do it? Instead of trying to make a person do what you want, why not find out what that person wants, then study your proposition to see what it has that will give him what he wants. Then show him how he can get what he wants by doing what you want. This is called motivation.

Chapter Eight
Help Others

When you try to convince a person to do what you want with no consideration for what he wants, that's manipulation.

What a person really wants depends on what is most important to him. What does he value most? What are his deepest needs and desires? He won't be very happy if he values something very much and ends up getting something else. Unless he is getting what he wants or what he values, he won't feel that he is achieving his outcome. It is important to all of us to become aware of what we want most; otherwise we won't end up getting it. Our values are usually emotional beliefs about something and they influence everything we do.

Your values were partly installed by your parents, teachers, and others who had influence over you in the early days of your life or by anyone or any situation which has a great impact on you at any stage in your life. For example, if you were raised in a very religious family and have strong religious convictions and a powerful desire to help others and convert them to your religious beliefs, you won't be very happy if you end up being a croupier in a gambling casino or a salesman of beer or wine or an entertainer in a striptease club.

Just as important as knowing your own values is knowing the values of your friends, associates, employees, relatives or anyone with whom you are associated or with whom you must cooperate.

Chapter Eight
Help Others

It is helpful to know the values of anyone whom you are trying to motivate. You will get people working for you only when you understand them and know what they really want. You will get them dedicated to working with you only if the job satisfies their values. Values are one of the most powerful motivational tools available to you.

Abraham Maslow, the founder of Humanistic Psychology, found that people on the job wanted security, belonging, recognition, satisfaction from achievement and the opportunity to grow and advance.

Some experts say that people want five things, some say twenty, and others say a hundred. It depends on how fine your classifications are. I believe the things that people want can be classified under twenty five headings and every person alive is struggling from the time they get up in the morning until they go to bed at night to get these twenty five things. These are the things they value. So when you try to persuade a person to do anything, you already know twenty five things that she wants. These twenty five things that constitute a person's hierarchy of values are the things we all value.

Here again is a list of the things that people want most. These are the conditions they value. You might try to find out which of these states is most important to you and this will help you to understand yourself better and know why you like and dislike

Chapter Eight
Help Others

certain situations and opportunities and even why you buy certain items.

1. To gain- money or material things
2. To save-security
3. Efficiency
4. To help others
5. Health
6. To think well of yourself
7. To have others think well of you
8. Creativity
9. Freedom
10. Sociability
11. Success
12. Excitment
13. Opportunity
15. Health
16. Peace of Mind
17. Power
18. Honesty
19. Loyalty
20. Teamwork
21. Love
23. Family
23. Sex
24. Peace of Mind
25. Physical activity

I think we can safely say that every person in the world is like every other person in that they want these twenty five things.

This is a way in which all people are alike and this gives us a rough guide to human behavior. We know that everyone wants all of these things. On the other hand, everyone in the world is completely different from everyone else in that he or she wants a different combination of these things. To some, freedom is the most important of these desired states, to others security or opportunity or the desire to think well of himself is most important. Once you know the combination of values that a

Chapter Eight
Help Others

person has you will understand him better and be in a better position to influence him. When you know your own sequence of values you will understand yourself better.

To gain money is one thing that men and women want and struggle for. Do you know anybody who doesn't want money? I don't. The newspapers report incidents of people who will rob to get it. Others will even kill to get it. Money is a very powerful motive. Sometimes when you are waiting in line at the bank you will notice someone who wants a loan so badly that he is wrestling the bank manager to the ground.

Yet we read about other men and women who don't want money as much as they want something else, even though they still need a certain amount of money to pay their basic expenses. Some men and women could make a fortune in certain fields of activity but prefer to dedicate their lives to helping others. Their big motive is not money. The thing they want most is to help people.

Albert Schweitzer was a great doctor, pianist and humanitarian. He could have made a financially successful career in several areas but he preferred to spend his life in Africa helping the sick and underprivileged.

Generally speaking, people want to help others. There is some of this drive in everybody. Don't underrate it. This is a motive

Chapter Eight
Help Others

for behavior that some of us overlook completely. Even the hard boiled business man has got some of this in him. The best example of this is the growth of the service clubs in the modern world. Kiwanis, Rotary, Lions and many other clubs have sprung up, and all are growing faster and getting bigger than ever. Why? Because most men and women at times examine themselves and say, "What am I contributing to the world?" and men and women will get together and devote their energies to helping the handicapped and underprivileged. And they grow and glow with this type of activity.

Ask yourself, "Is there anything in my proposition that will enable this person to help others? If so, I might be able to persuade him". Most people from time to time do things to help others. The businessman, for example, will sometimes buy a new computer, not because he wants one but because he thinks it will be good for his secretary. Or he might install air conditioning in his office if it will help his staff to be more comfortable and enjoy their work more.

What about saving and protecting? I don't know anybody who doesn't want security. All the people I know are planning for their security with insurance policies, pension plans, etc. Why? To be secure. To make sure money is not only coming in today but that it is going to continue to be there in the future.

Chapter Eight
Help Others

Some people are more security minded than others. Some men and women hoard their money, depriving themselves of things they need today because they had a rough experience during the last depression and don't want to be in that position again. If you have anything in your proposition that will bring this type of person security you will have a good chance of convincing him.

Every person wants to be efficient. People are buying computers, cell phones and hiring people to maintain their lawn, remove their snow and anything that will bring more efficiency and pleasure into their lives. There is a strong drive in the human make-up to do things efficiently. If you have anything in the idea you are trying to put across that will make the other person more efficient, don't hesitate to mention it. If you are trying to influence your son to buy a personal computer you can tell him about the pleasure he will get from the things he can do on the computer. But you may have a better chance of influencing him by telling him how efficient he will become in his studies and at his work if he uses a computer.

Pleasure is something that everybody wants. A basic drive in everyone is the drive to feel good. More and more money is being spent on travel, sports and entertainment than ever before. People are going all out to try and enjoy life. You can appeal to this motive in almost anyone you are trying to persuade.

Chapter Eight
Help Others

Every man and woman wants to think well of himself or herself. You may call it pride. If you have anything in your idea that will help the person to think better of himself, he will be interested. There aren't enough policemen in the world to police all of us. If we were all criminals in tendency, it would be impossible for us to live together. We would be robbing and stealing. Fortunately, most people have a little policeman inside themselves who says, "How could you live with yourself if you did that?" With some people the little policeman goes off duty at times.

Part of pride is the desire to impress others favorably and to gain recognition. We all spend much energy to try and get people to admire and respect us. From the time you get up in the morning till you go to bed at night, just about everything you do is slanted towards impressing people.

Maybe the best example of someone trying to impress others is the man who buys a very expensive car although he can't afford it. He buys it because when he drives down the street, he thinks people will look at him and say, "Look at that smart fellow go!" Although he may impress some people, others think he is suffering with delusions of grandeur. Have you got anything in your idea that will enable the person you are trying to convince to impress others favorably or to gain recognition?

Chapter Eight
Help Others

Most people would like to be very creative so they can make wise decisions and be able to create new and better ways of doing things. Others are keenly interested in the artistic type of creativity where they can paint, write, or compose music. If your needs are strong in the creative area and your job doesn't satisfy this need, try to develop a hobby or part time activity in which you can use your creativity. If you are trying to persuade someone to do something, they may become creative in ways to avoid doing what you want them to.

Freedom or independence is the most important value to some people. They would prefer a job with less money in which they can be their own boss to a higher paid job where they must work under supervision. Working on their own with complete authority and responsibility is worth more to this type of person than money. Is there anything in the idea that you are promoting which will enable a person to have more freedom?

For some people, socializing with others is all important. They need to work in a setting where people are involved. They like being part of a team, so it is important if you are trying to convince her to do something to mention that your idea will bring her into contact with others.

How about satisfaction from achievement? Do you know anybody who doesn't want to do their work better? Most people I

Chapter Eight
Help Others

know are reading technical journals, taking night school courses, correspondence courses, subscribing to magazines, or reading new books, trying to keep up to date and develop themselves so they can achieve their goals. The thrill of having knowledge, doing well, and achieving is to many people the greatest satisfaction of all.

Is there something in your idea that will give a person opportunity to advance? If so, it will help you to persuade that person. Some men and women want opportunity. It could be something that will give the person a specialized type of knowledge or greater skill which will improve his opportunity to advance.

Everybody wants good health. Most of the people I know are dieting, exercising, taking vitamins and practising a certain regimen to gain better health. This has become a powerful motive in the last few years because of the tremendous death toll from cancer, heart disease and strokes. If you have anything in your idea that will help a person to improve his health, mention it, no matter how small it might be: it might be the thing that convinces him. Don't underrate the possibility of an improvement in mental health. If you can ease the daily pressure on a person and make life easier for him or her, this will certainly be of interest. Many people realize that good health is more important than impressing people or making money.

Chapter Eight
Help Others

Thinking and reasoning are very important to certain people. The universities are filled with professors and researchers who have no great ambitions to make money or impress others but they like to think and reason at a high level. To them thinking is stimulating and exciting. If you are trying to convince a person who places high value on thinking, you must show him how your proposition will give him this opportunity.

Peace of mind is one of the most important of all the values. How can you enjoy life if you don't have peace of mind? If you don't feel right about yourself and your relationships with others, nothing else really matters. Some people are rich in money but riddled with guilt and fear because of their immoral or dishonest dealings and they go through life in constant turmoil and distress. Feeling good or having peace of mind is the ultimate goal for everyone although each person has a different way to achieve this outcome.

Do you know anyone who likes to have power? Feeling in control of situations and people is important to people who like power. They work hard to accumulate wealth and build big corporations. Not always because they want to make money but to have people under their control. He loves the power of hiring and firing and controlling the destinies of others. Is there anything in your proposition that will give a person power? If so, talk about it.

Chapter Eight
Help Others

Loyalty, honesty, team work and love are important to all of us. So are family, sex, companionship, excitement and physical activity. So be sure and mention anything in your proposition that will bring a person any of these needs.

I have given you twenty-five powerful keys to persuading people. Any of these values could enable you to persuade a person if you can prove that your idea will produce the benefit for the person involved. And all you have to do when you try to persuade or motivate somebody is say, "I have an idea that will help you to improve your health," or similar words that describe one of the twenty-five things that people want. She will probably say, "I'm skeptical. I don't believe it, but I'll listen. Tell me about it." Then if you can prove to her that she will get one or more of these twenty-five things by doing what you are suggesting, she will probably do it.

Every man or woman is exactly like every other man or woman in that they want these twenty-five things. And yet every individual is completely different from every other individual because he or she wants a different combination of these twenty-five things.

Keep asking, what is of most interest to her. A person will frequently reveal her most important values by saying, "If you had something that would help me to cut my expenses, I'd be

Chapter Eight
Help Others

interested." Then you know that saving or protecting is one of her important values.

After you have talked to a person who agrees that your idea will do everything you say, she may still not accept your proposition. Why? Because everybody is indecisive. Decision making is difficult. Some of us of course, are more indecisive than others. Because decision making is dangerous. It's gambling, it's risk taking. Every time a person agrees to something different she is taking a chance, or she may be making a mistake by taking this action.

There is no easy way to get a person to make a decision, but one of the best ways is to ask him to do what it is you want him to do. For example, if a married woman is trying to persuade her husband to take up the game of golf to improve his health, she could say, "Will you do something about this right now and buy yourself a set of golf clubs?" sometimes just asking helps a person to make up his mind. Otherwise he might think about it, but do nothing. Some wives whose husbands are dedicated golfers have to ask the reverse questions, "Will you take action and destroy those golf clubs right now or will you find a new wife?"

The asking of questions is also a good way to nudge a person towards agreement with you. Questions have been called, "the levers of thought." By questioning you can sometimes influence

Chapter Eight
Help Others

a person's thoughts; since thoughts control actions, questions can often influence action.

Questions can be the dynamic forces of persuasion. By asking questions you can reason together. Try to find something that you can agree on in a situation where you are trying to persuade someone and then question them in this area. In the case of a wife trying to get her husband to take up golf she might ask, "Do you agree that the fresh air and sunshine would be good for you?" this is something he would have to agree with and from there they might reason together and finally he may be convinced.

When a person presents a new idea to someone the natural reaction of the other person is to say, "No, I can't do that" instead, if you talk about one of the twenty-five things everybody wants, he or she has to be interested.

If you are trying to persuade your husband to take up the game of golf because his doctor ordered him to get more exercise you might talk to him about how it will improve his health, enable him to enjoy life more, and live longer and get him out of the house more before you strangle him. You might also show him how by becoming more relaxed, he will become more efficient at his work and make more money on the job. You might tell him that others will be impressed with his new activity. He may also meet important people through his new activity that could help

Chapter Eight
Help Others

him in many ways. Don't urge him to take up the game of golf but try to show him how golf will give him some of the twenty-five things he wants in life.

You must be careful in any persuasive action you are taking not to set up a competitive situation where you are trying to persuade the other person of something and they are trying not to be persuaded. This could lead to an argument where both parties are trying to win their point without giving any thought to the other person's point of view. This sometimes ends in tempers flaring and hostilities being aroused.

To prevent this, try to find something in the situation on which you seem to agree and then ask questions in that area to establish some common ground of agreement. For example, you may be arguing with someone who supports socialism as a way of life, while you support the free enterprise system. You might ask the question, "Is it fair to say that we are both searching for the same thing but in different ways, and that you want the maximum benefits for all the people and I want the same thing?" From that common ground, you may then ask more questions and avoid an emotional confrontation.

In some arguments, both parties are basically in agreement, but because of the hostility involved they do not understand the other person's point of view. A good way to prevent this from

Chapter Eight
Help Others

happening is to insist that when one person has expressed his point of view, the other person is required to repeat what he said but using different words. In this way, the first person will be able to clarify what he really meant. If each party is required to clearly state the other person's viewpoint to his or her satisfaction, this forces each to see and understand the other's position.

As you become expert in the techniques of persuasion, you will be able to discover the elements in any proposition that will satisfy some of the twenty-five values of each person. Then you will be able to convince people to do things. Persuading others will then be a psychological game which will be interesting, stimulating and challenging and will be a great assist in helping you to keep in a good mental state. It will relieve frustration and discouragement when you are blocked in trying to convince someone of something.

Knowledge of how to convince and persuade people will make life smoother and make you feel good. You will get real satisfaction from convincing your family and your friends to do things that will be good for them and will make them healthier, happier and more effective. Constantly feeling good has much to do with moving through life free of tension and frustration. To do this, it's important to be able to get along with others and be able to persuade them to do things.

Chapter Eight
Help Others

Sometimes you will have difficulty in getting along with others because you have an opinion and you stick to it in spite of the fact that your partner, friend or lover is giving you strong evidence that your position is not right. The desire to be right and to prove that you know best is often an emotional position that you take and stick to with stubborn determination.

At this point you should ask yourself, "would you rather be right or would you rather be happy?" Often you may stick to a position just to prove that you know best. The result is to keep yourself in a weak state. Instead why not say, "That's an interesting viewpoint. Tell me more about why you feel you are right about this." There are some people, of course, who would rather be right than happy.

People with good mental health get along well with others because they have respect for them. If you treat another with respect, you will gain his respect. If you don't get along well with others, they will criticize you and hurt you and put you in a poor mental state.

The other big way in which getting along with others can help you to feel good is that friends can be a great support when you have problems. If you have a close friend who will listen to your problems, this can often be as helpful as going to a psychiatrist. What the psychiatrist can do for you is hold up his listening

Chapter Eight
Help Others

mirror. When he listens to you and gets you talking, you begin to see yourself in his listening mirror and often when you see what you are really like, you will get enough insight into your problem that you can cure yourself. A wise friend can do the same thing,

The other thing the psychiatrist does is to reassure you that you are a worthwhile person no matter what you have done in the past. This can be a great relief if you have been blaming and criticizing yourself for certain things you have done which you believe are terrible things. The psychiatrist will reassure you that these things aren't terrible, that practically everybody is doing them and that you are OK no matter what you have done. A good friend can do the same thing. Having a close friend is like having a psychiatrist available all the time. This will help you to keep feeling good most of the time.

Life Line Exercise

To get your subconscious mind working for you in human relations, I suggest you move out into your immediate future in your life line and create a picture of yourself getting along well with a group of people and acting like a natural leader. Get right into this picture and notice what you see, what you hear and how you feel. Enjoy all of these sensations in relating to the people around you. Turn up the brightness and make the scene more colorful, clearly focused and larger. Put more

Chapter Eight
Help Others

movement in it. Now at the peak of your enjoyment, step out of this picture and hang it on your life line while you watch yourself making friends and getting along well with others.

By placing this picture on your life line, you are motivating your subconscious mind to move towards making you the kind of person you have visualized in this picture. By putting it on your life line, you can see yourself in this picture any time. This will keep reinforcing this new image which you want to create.

Here is your conditioning statement on human relations. Whenever you have a problem with anyone or have a problem getting along with someone, keep repeating this statement over and over. Repeat it several times on waking in the morning and before going to bed at night:

I understand people, I like people and I can motivate others and get along well with them.

The Good Book of Godliness
Notes

Chapter Nine

Develop Your Interests

How would you feel if you could suddenly play par golf or if you won the club championship of your tennis club or your softball team won the league championship? Or if you won a bridge, checkers, chess or ping-pong tournament? If achievement of any kind moves you into a great state, go and do something at which you can create, learn, achieve, meet people, develop a skill, travel or help someone with a problem so you will feel good right now.

Remember the day you finished building your summer cottage, or you took your first solo flight in an airplane or your department was awarded a prize for being the best in your company or you became top salesperson in your organization or you were elected president of a social club? Any of these things could make you feel good.

Fill your life with activities at which you can win, achieve, learn, develop your skills, create, meet new people, travel and help

Chapter Nine
Develop Your Interests

people with their problems. These activities will help you to keep feeling good.

Wide interests also enable you to relax. When you are tired you may not need a rest, you may need a change of pace. Wisdom comes from wide interests that bring you into contact with many people and many different situations from which you learn. Wider interests also help you in getting along better with others. Who do you like best, a person who is sitting at home staring into space or one who is active and doing interesting things? Another advantage of wide interests is that you become more creative. Usually creative action comes about because you have adapted some idea from one of your experiences. Those with wider interests have more experiences to draw from.

Wider interests, of course, improve your mental health. The more activities in which you participate, the more sources of satisfaction you have and the more emotional support you have in adjusting to the adversities of life. If one activity is eliminated, you still have several other satisfying ways to spend your time. Each successful activity in which you invest your time brings you eustress, which gives you enthusiasm for your other activities.

Abraham Maslow, the father of Humanistic Psychology has said that to get to be happy we must each do everything we are capable of doing. In other words, to lead a full life and feel good we must

Chapter Nine
Develop Your Interests

each use all of our talents to the fullest. Life is a struggle to find our talents and use them.

The development of good mental health begins in childhood. Babies are not born neurotic; babies don't worry. They learn how to worry as they grow up. When a child is born he is completely dependent on his parents to feed him, clothe him and keep him warm. As he matures, he struggles to become independent of his parents. He does this by substituting dependence on activities in his life and on other people, for dependence on his parents. As time goes by, he gains the contacts and skills necessary to feel good without his parents.

First he gets to associate with and depend on his own friends. At school he soon gets interested in academic subjects. Then he gets active in sports. This draws him away from his parents some more. Next he develops a hobby, perhaps collecting stamps. Eventually he discovers a philosophy of life and starts to believe in something bigger than himself. Then he gets a job in which he becomes absorbed. Finally he falls in love and creates a family of his own, which puts him in the best state of all.

The person who fails to develop adequate supports to replace his parents is in danger of falling into a weak state, and he may also drive his parents to the psychiatrist. The truth is that nobody is capable of being completely independent. We all need supports

Chapter Nine
Develop Your Interests

to keep feeling good. To help you to find the right kinds of activities that will bring you satisfaction from achievement and independence, I suggest that you go over your life history and try to recall anything you did at any time of your life which you enjoyed doing, did well and about which you felt good. Don't concern yourself about the situation in which you did these things. It could have been as a hobby or in your academic or sports life or at your work. As long as you enjoyed it, did it well and felt good about it, start doing it again. Things you like doing are like diamonds in the rough, pounce on them and keep doing them over and over.

Undoubtedly you can recall a time when you were feeling depressed. Perhaps you had been invited to a party but the last thing you wanted to do was go to one. However, you forced yourself to go and later you found you were quite exhilarated by the contacts with others, the stimulating interchange of ideas and the challenge of making new friends. This put you in a better state. Your depression was reduced by the time you got home. People contacts have a positive effect on your state. The person who is socially active is more likely to feel good and enjoy life than a person who keeps to himself.

At another time, you may have been worried about something, but you plunged headlong into your favorite hobby of woodworking, stamp collecting, bricklaying, scuba diving, golf or mountain

Chapter Nine
Develop Your Interests

climbing. After a few hours of participation in the activity you most enjoyed, you felt more relaxed and in a better state. Perhaps you even found that your problem had been resolved by your subconscious mind.

A hobby should be something you enjoy doing. It must not be a chore. It should be an escape from day to day routine, an activity in which you can totally lose yourself. This type of activity gives you satisfaction from achievement, which will change your state and give you good feelings. It doesn't matter what your hobby is, as long as you find it interesting, absorbing, and rewarding. Anything at which you can achieve, learn, create, develop a skill, meet new people or help people with their problems will put you in a state that will make you feel good and stimulate you to take actions, to solve your problems.

Sports are ideal as a hobby. Sports offer an outlet for tension and excess energy and also contribute to body conditioning. Game sports in particular provide a challenge because of the competition involved. The "team spirit" alone may change your state and give you energy. Playing the game will also bring you satisfaction which helps to make you feel good.

The body thrives on physical challenge and the mind thrives on mental challenge. For this reason I believe that every person should have some type of academic interest in his life. We all need

Chapter Nine
Develop Your Interests

something to challenge our minds, some intellectual stimulation that goes beyond selecting the right necktie. So pick some field like mathematics, history, psychology, philosophy, anthropology, geography, astronomy and start to do some studying. Either take a night school course at your local university or go to the library and start a reading program in some area of interest.

Not only will this develop your mind and put you in a new state, but it will also widen your interests and thereby help to make you wiser and more creative. George Bernard Shaw said that he found thinking so stimulating that it was more pleasurable than sex. This indicates what powerful satisfaction thinking can bring to some and what an exalted state it can put them in. My advice is to get some kind of mental challenge going for you so you will have another way to get yourself feeling good.

Naturally a happy home life contributes much to your happiness. You have probably had the experience of a particularly difficult day at the office, which depressed you and irritated you. That night you came home to your wife and children, or your parents or brothers or sisters or your roommate, feeling miserable. You felt like biting everyone in sight. But after some bantering conversation and griping on your part, for which you probably received support and consolation, you were feeling better.

Chapter Nine
Develop Your Interests

The key to a secure and harmonious family life is to always practice good human relations with people close to you. Don't be tactless, hostile, demanding and unfeeling. Keep alert and be friendly, thoughtful and sympathetic and you will find your family responding to you. If you have someone in the family who will listen to your problems in an understanding manner, this is like having a psychiatrist right at home. Often all you need to solve your problems is someone to listen, sympathize and let you know that you are accepted as you are with all your hang-ups and limitations. This will change your state and give you the power to solve your own problems. You can reciprocate by listening to your partner's problems and sympathizing with your partner and reassuring him/her that what he or she is doing is not all that bad.

The problem with some marriages or relationships is that the partners are congenial and friendly with strangers but complaining, critical, and demanding with one another. They put on a great act when out socially but at home where they should be pleasant, they complain and criticize. If they treated the mailman like they treat their wives, he would stop delivering the mail.

People could not live together in harmony if they didn't have work to challenge and satisfy them. A job that you like and do well is important. Earning money is a necessity in our modern

Chapter Nine
Develop Your Interests

society, but more important is to find work that offers you an opportunity to utilize your skills, talents, initiative and drive.

For a healthy balance, the right job should challenge you, give you an opportunity to advance and keep you striving, yet not be so difficult that it sends you home frustrated at the end of each day or ready to be carried home on a stretcher. Ideally you should enjoy your job because of the actual work you are doing, not because of the power, prestige, or financial rewards. A person who is striving to do his job well will get satisfaction from achievement and feel good.

Although money should never become the most important reason for living, having some money in the bank will make you more secure and put you in a better state. Try to live within your means and save a little. Avoid gambling and taking financial risks: losing money could distress you and put you in a poor state. Money may not always bring happiness, but a lack of money can certainly bring you unhappiness. If you don't have enough to buy food, clothing and shelter, you will be very unhappy. Accumulating a lot of money, however, has limitations for making you exceptionally happy. A man with ten million dollars is just as happy as a man with eleven million dollars.

Money is more than the means of buying necessities. It is a symbol of your success. If you live in a mansion and drive a Rolls-Royce,

Chapter Nine
Develop Your Interests

you are signalling to the world that you are a smart person to have been able to master your environment and yourself and other people to the degree that you have been able to accumulate many markers (dollars) that indicate the degree of your smartness.

How happy you will be with much money depends on yourself. Once you have provided for your basic security, it will depend on your make-up. If you are a show off and lacking in self esteem, you will need lots of symbols to prove to the world that you are a worthwhile person. If you have high self esteem, you won't need to bolster your confidence with exotic material possessions.

The answer is to accumulate enough money to give you security and peace of mind but don't sacrifice your integrity or your reputation to gain more symbols of success. It may not make you happier. Don't base your happiness and peace of mind on accumulating wealth. You will never be satisfied. The more you make, the more you will want. There is no end to the accumulation of material things that will satisfy you. You will find men and women in the world who have hundreds of millions of dollars who are still striving for more.

Traveling can excite and stimulate you. Experiencing a foreign country gives you a feeling of being alive. You feel youthful while traveling because you are exploring, playing, being spontaneous and adventuresome. It brings out new things in yourself when

Chapter Nine
Develop Your Interests

you explore the newness of a foreign country or travel to distant points in your own country.

Traveling is therapeutic because it takes you away from stressful situations and gets you concentrating on the present environment. The problems of arranging accommodation, transportation and making sure you get to see the important sights are so great that you are forced to forget your problems and live in the present. You won't worry about your telephone bill while floating through Venice on a gondola.

Sometimes you face the challenge of loneliness in a new country without friends, home and your usual supports. This builds inner strength. When you travel you are also learning. You are observing new lifestyles, you are hearing new languages and you are learning the history and geography of the places you are visiting.

Mentally healthy people are active and productive. They use their abilities and resources on their own behalf and to help others. One of the most effective ways to feel good is to help underprivileged people. You will feel useful and purposeful when you work with handicapped children or teach a skill and bring some enjoyment to others. Try to become actively involved. A donation is helpful in support of a charity or cultural organization, but it won't do you as much good as actual participation. If you get personally involved in helping people solve their problems you will tend to

Chapter Nine
Develop Your Interests

forget your own problems. If you are always helping others you won't have time to worry about your own problems.

Faith in something bigger than yourself is another important support to keep you in a good mental state. Religious faith or belief in God is one of the most important ways to keep feeling good. Those who believe in God have constant spiritual support. This faith will put them in a state to bear adverse conditions and will also give them the strength to widen their interests and participate in varied activities.

Mentally healthy people substitute activities in many areas for their original dependence on parents. They participate in a wide variety of activities that make life interesting for them and keep them in a good state. If one avenue becomes closed, they have many others to follow. If they are only active in three areas, it is like a car running on three cylinders. However, it's more important to develop a good quality of activity in a few areas than to rush into many fields of endeavour and master none.

A good state is not a static position that you can achieve and then relax. You can never say, "Now I am happy and I can stop working on it." To keep in a healthy mental state is elusive, but it is there for you in all areas of your life. It is the constant pursuit of a better state that is likely to bring you closest to it.

Chapter Nine
Develop Your Interests

When you undertake any activity, try to do it in an excellent manner. When you do something really well, you get satisfaction from achievement or eustress. This will carry over into everything you do. For example, if you paint pictures as a hobby and get very good at what you are creating, this will put you in a state of mind so you will become a better worker, a better friend, a better father or mother and a better all round person.

If you excel in academic achievement the eustress from this will make you a better painter, better student, etc. When you have activities in several areas of your life, the eustress from each of these will combine to give you a synergistic effect and lift you into a very powerful state. In my book Synergy and the Power of Personal Proficiency (Hunter Carlyle Publishing, 1983) I have outlined how wider interests bring synergy and energy into your life.

You will hear frequently from the experts that your bad states aren't caused by the conditions you face but by your attitude toward those conditions. This is true. However, don't kid yourself, the better the circumstances in which you live the easier it will be for you to feel good. Facing adversity and coming up positive isn't easy but it will develop your character and your personal strengths.

Life is a struggle to achieve, get along with others and be happy. To do these things you need to be active. You must keep monitoring

Chapter Nine
Develop Your Interests

your activities and when you feel in a bad state from a lack of action, take on more things, on the other hand, if you feel stress from too much action, cut back on some things you are doing.

Life Line Exercise

Fly out over your life line in your imagination to a place about one year in the future. Visualize yourself talking to some friends who are asking you how you got interested in the arts, social service, academic, sports and social activities. Get right into this picture. Note what your friends are wearing and what they are saying and concentrate on how good it feels to have many things going for you. Brighten this picture, make it bigger, clearer, moving, and more colorful and bring it in closer or whatever gives it more impact for you. When you are feeling at your best in this picture, step out of it and hang it on your life line while you are watching yourself in the picture. Now fly back to the present.

Put other pictures in your life line of you participating in the arts, sports, academic, social service, social or whatever areas of interest you have.

Here is a statement to use constantly to help you to widen your interests. Keep saying this in a strong positive voice with feeling and it will get through to your subconscious mind:

Chapter Nine
Develop Your Interests

My interests are wide, which makes me wiser and more creative and helps me to get along better with people and have better mental health.

Notes

Notes

Chapter Ten

Join

Join or join in... one of the greatest pleasures I enjoy are the clubs I have joined over the years. I am a member of the Arts and Letters Club, Rotary Club of Toronto, Rosedale Golf Club, Royal Canadian Yacht Club, and the Granite Club. These clubs have not only helped me spiritually but have helped in my business as well.

Not everyone can afford to join clubs but there are plenty of alternatives that don't cost money. Organize a group for walking each day. This will not only help you continue to be fit but will also give you the companionship of people like yourself. Use this time to bounce ideas off your colleagues and in return you can also be of service to them and their challenges.

Go to the YMCA or join a book club through your local library. Volunteer! There are many associations, schools, nursing homes that would thrilled to have an extra pair of hands in organizing

Chapter Ten
Join

and helping. There are many ways to join or join in that don't cost money.

Offer to help your neighbor by walking their dog or help them with their gardening.

Notes

Notes

Chapter Eleven

Knowledge

Knowledge is a wonderful thing. The more you learn the bigger your world becomes.

Read at least one new thing each day and not just the newspaper, which can be filled with negativity and problems. Go to the library (the one you just joined for free) and find books in which you are interested. Reading things that interest you will get you more involved with the information. Once you have started you won't be able to hold yourself back.

Take the dictionary and learn at least two new words a week. Then write them in sentences so it resonates with you. If two words are too much, learn one a week. This will expand your vocabulary and help you express yourself in different ways.

There are many television programs now that offer you a variety of interesting topics to learn about. The Discovery Channel is a

Chapter Eleven
Knowledge

good example or you can go to the video store and rent different series of programs on all sorts of topics. The library also has a large selection of videos you can borrow so you don't have to spend the money.

Words are important because we think with words. The larger your vocabulary the wider your thinking will be and eventually this will widen your interests and activities.

Keep expanding your knowledge base and soon you will have new and different interests and along with that will come new friends.

Notes

Chapter Twelve

Laugh

Laugh and the world laughs with you because laughing puts everyone in a good state. Laugh as much as you can. How can you get yourself to laugh right now? It's easy. Just create an artificial laugh. Just chant "ha ha ha – ha ha ha – ha ha ha" and your state will begin to change. Keep up this artificial laugh and smile while you are doing it. Stand straight and look up. Keep moving around and visualize yourself being happy and joyful and you should eliminate your feelings of distress.

Think of one of the funniest incidents you can remember. Try to get the feeling of that humorous situation. Visualize yourself right back in that incident and in a great humorous state. Think of what you saw and heard and how you felt on that occasion. How were you standing or sitting? Make the picture brighter, clearer more colorful, larger and move it in close to yourself. Reproduce your posture and what you saw, heard and felt. Now at the height of your humorous feeling take a deep breath and

Chapter Twelve
Laugh

go "ha ha ha – ha ha ha – ha ha ha" and at the same time press your thumbs against your forefingers. Linger mentally in this humorous situation and do your artificial laugh several times with your thumbs and forefingers pressing together. You should now be anchored to this joyous situation and you should be able to bring this feeling back anytime by visualizing it and going "ha ha ha – ha ha ha – ha ha ha" and pressing your thumbs and forefingers together. Try it. If it doesn't work the first time, keep trying. Keep laughing and smiling and you will be happy.

Have you ever been in a depressed mood and then somebody made a humorous comment or a funny joke and suddenly you broke into laughing and into a new state of mind and body? It happened immediately. Or have you ever been in a solemn group where there is some conflict and it looks as if things are turning into a fighting situation and someone suddenly makes a humorous comment and in a flash everyone starts to laugh and immediately everyone is in a better state of mind.

Laughing and smiling are two of the fastest ways to eliminate distress. So I am going to explore with you some of the ways you can use laughter to change states quickly. I will also look into the possibility of using humour in your life to constantly keep you free of distress.

Chapter Twelve
Laugh

Comedians earn fabulous incomes because they can take a group of tired, worried business men or women and suddenly change their state and get them smiling and laughing. The highest paid entertainers in the world are paid all that money because they can make people laugh. Humorous books, movies and TV shows are great tools for eliminating distress.

People with a sense of humour who can bring fun and laughter into almost any situation are the most popular people because we all want to improve our states of mind and we welcome anyone who can help us do it. Men who have the most success with women are those who can make them laugh. When a woman starts to laugh she changes state, feels good and looks favorably on the man who can do it. In the human relations area, laughter is one of the best techniques for getting along with people of both sexes and gaining their support. A woman with a sense of humour is desirable to a man because when she gets him laughing, she eliminates his distress.

In the public speaking business, the best communicators are those who mix their serious comments with funny lines. People like to laugh because it eliminates their distress. They like to be entertained while they are learning. The highest paid speakers are humorists as well as educators.

Chapter Twelve
Laugh

Are you enjoying life? How much pleasure are you getting out of life? These are the first questions I would ask you to determine your state and your mental health.

How much you laugh and smile will tell if all is well. It will tell me if you are enjoying life and feeling good. These are the clues that indicate you are free of distress and depression. If you are unhappy and worried about something and are suffering with distress I can change this if I can get you laughing and smiling.

Because the main symptom of mental ill health is unhappiness, worry and depression, it seems to me the front line of attack against mental ill health should be to try and keep happy. Let's put it this way; when you start to over-worry and get depressed, this is a signal that something is wrong. You are either doing something that is unhealthy or you are thinking in a way that distresses you

You can do much to bring more fun and humour into your life by anchoring yourself to humorous situations and by using your "ha ha ha – ha ha ha – ha ha ha" and thumbs pressing on forefingers to recall these humorous states. You can also bring more humour into your life by visualizing yourself as a humorous person. Another way to become more humorous is to get your subconscious mind slanted in a humorous direction.

Chapter Twelve
Laugh

The fist step towards seeing the humorous side of things and enjoying life is to understand that with all the different types of people in the world and the many different situations we have to face, there are bound to be some unusual things happen.

Don't expect too much too soon from life and you won't be disappointed when things don't work out exactly as you planned. Don't take yourself and life too seriously. It's a game. Play it as well as you can, but don't expect to be perfect or even near perfect. You win some and you lose some as you go through life.

Nothing is more important than laughter in your growth and development. When you are laughing, it's nature's signal that you are in a good state, making progress and free of distress. Experiencing pleasure is a very positive feeling. It gives you strength to do all the things you must do for success. It makes you more confident and helps you to think well of yourself. It enables you to appreciate life and all its blessings. It keeps you in a good state.

Humour is found in an imperfect world. Laughter and humour are ways of dealing with the world's shortcomings.

I urge you to get pleasure from doing things and achieving, learning, creating, developing your skills, travelling, meeting new people, and helping people with their problems. Doing

Chapter Twelve
Laugh

these things will put you in a good state. Relaxing, meditating, philosophizing and day-dreaming can also improve your state.

These inner pleasures can be just as great as the pleasures that come from activities.

Unfortunately, many people are unable to enjoy fully the joys of living. They may have been trained to reject pleasure and have been taught to take responsibility too seriously, to keep their noses to the grindstone and work hard. They may have been taught that having fun is a frivolous waste of time. If only they knew that fun and laughter and pleasure can sometimes save their lives by relieving distress and helping them to roll with the punches, and enjoy the simple pleasures in the present.

Many people who are striving to be rich and famous are unhappy because they are always looking forward to the day when they will have more money or be prime minister or president. There is nothing wrong with being ambitious, but there are many things wrong with passing up present joy and pleasure for an uncertain future.

In our day-to-day struggle to survive and make a living, we have tended to become too serious. The grim pursuit of work and the difficulties of getting the job done have absorbed many of us so much that we have put laughter, pleasure, having fun and

Chapter Twelve
Laugh

enjoying life on the back burner. The pursuit of achievement, power, skill, money and status has taken over and we are in a more serious state than nature intended and can easily suffer with distress.

The original man and woman in the jungle was a playful, fun loving person who had to struggle to eat and survive but their capacity to play and laugh and enjoy life kept them in a relaxed state gave them relief from distress, fear and insecurity. They didn't return home to their cave with ulcers because other cavemen had collected more bananas than they did. Playing and laughing were a very important part of life in the jungle.

Animals know how to play and relax by gamboling, stretching and dozing in the sun. They get real pleasure from their present environment, which puts them in a great state. They don't worry or fret about past events or have heated arguments with their stockbrokers.

Action always comes first. If you want to be confident, act confident and you will eventually be confident. If you want to be happy, act happy. If you want to enjoy life, act as if you are enjoying it, so sing, whistle, and laugh whenever you can. Keep using your artificial laugh "ha ha ha – ha ha ha – ha ha ha" and press your thumbs and forefingers together and visualize yourself in a happy situation free of distress.

Chapter Twelve
Laugh

There is much evidence that fun, humour and laughter affect not only our mental health but our physical health. Throughout history, the great thinkers and philosophers have been telling us that humour and laughter are therapeutic. Freud said that humour was a good way to counteract nervous tension. Emmanuel Kant said that laughter produces a feeling of good health and stimulates the body processes.

Probably our best example of how effective laughter can be in the health area comes from Norman Cousins, author of *Anatomy of an Illness* (Bantam Books). In his book, he describes how he helped cure himself of an apparently incurable physical disease by thinking positively and laughing as much as possible.

Unfortunately, humour which triggers laughter is very difficult to generate. We continue to tell the same old jokes with variations, and comedians steal jokes and funny situations from one another, because to produce humour is a very difficult task. Will Rogers, Stephen Leacock, Woody Allen, James Thurber, Mark Twain, Dorothy Parker, Groucho Marx and a few other writers and performer have been able to create original humour and we revere them for this rare talent. Bob Hope, George Burns, Bill Cosby, Eddie Murphy, Red Skelton, Johnny Carson and many other comedians have become rich because our society is willing to pay a big price in order to laugh.

Chapter Twelve
Laugh

Let me alert you to some of the benefits that can come to you from laughing. Physiologically, laughing stimulates your blood circulation and exercises your lungs. It also exercises your diaphragm, which is a muscle between your chest and your stomach. If you put your hand on your stomach while you are laughing, you will feel the diaphragm moving up and down, exercising the muscles in this area of your body.

When you laugh, it causes you to breathe more deeply and take more oxygen into your blood. The entire heart-lung-blood delivery system benefits when you laugh. Laughter is very relaxing to your body as well as to your mind and emotions. When you laugh at something, you forget your problems, at least temporarily.

The experts tell us that laughter produces endorphins in the brain which reduce pain. When you laugh you get a new slant on life because you become less intense, more objective and not so deeply involved.

To feel good and be happy is one of the greatest needs of human beings.

Some great thinkers have said that the purpose of life is to feel good. Feeling good is an indication that your life is going well and you are in a good state. Having pleasure and enjoying life and laughing may be the secrets of success. this is why successful

Chapter Twelve
Laugh

people tend to be fun-loving people. When I first discovered this, I thought that these people were happy because they were successful. But I later found that they were probably successful because they were happy.

Laughing and having fun stimulates the pituitary gland, which has an influence on your energy and vitality, so necessary to success. Enjoyment and pleasure will stimulate you and put you in a relaxed state. So laugh as much as possible. Search out things that bring you pleasure and be as active as possible in these things. Start to enjoy yourself right now. Begin with the simple pleasures of developing skills, reading, learning, visiting with friends, walking in the country and enjoying the beauty of nature.

Some writers have declared laughter to be beneficial because it restores homeostasis, stabilizing blood pressure, oxygenating the blood, massaging the vital organs, stimulating circulation, facilitating digestion, relaxing the system and producing a feeling of well being.

In spite of these physical changes that take place when you laugh, I am sure that the psychological and emotional changes are just as important. The playful attitude that encompasses you and the resulting relaxation are the most therapeutic actions you could take for relieving distress. You can't be suffering from distress

Chapter Twelve
Laugh

when you are laughing. Try to worry and laugh at the same time. It's impossible.

To me this means that we should take action in our lives, which will bring us pleasure and cause us to smile or laugh. If successful mentally healthy people are happy people who enjoy fun and laughing, one of the best routes to success and happiness is to search for all the things in your life that you like to do, that you do well and that make you feel good and give you pleasure. Spend as much time doing these things as you can so you will enjoy life and laugh as much as possible.

Another way to get a laugh is with the humorous catalogue. This is a situation where you have a list of items to which you add an item at the end of the list that is unexpected and out of context. For example. I might say that he is a great golfer because he has a smooth swing, putts accurately, chips and pitches with precision and he can't add. The last item is out of context and unexpected and will get a smile or a snicker or a belly laugh depending on who you are telling it to.

So keep watching for situations where you can exaggerate, understate, suddenly change the train of through or create a humourous catalogue and you should be able to create some humour as you go your daily rounds. Of course there are other ways but these are the best. Create humour to amuse yourself

Chapter Twelve
Laugh

and get into the habit of seeing the fun in life. Don't expect many brilliantly funny lines. Creating humour is very difficult. If you can do it easily and effortlessly, you may become rich.

When you awaken each morning, if you have trouble swinging into action, sit on the side of your bed and reproduce your artificial laugh in order to get your day started right. Go "ha ha ha – ha ha ha – ha ha ha" and press your thumbs and forefingers together. This will do several things for you. First it will start some of the positive physical and psychological activities in your body that are triggered by laughing and give you a toning effect. It will also alert you to the fact that you shouldn't take life or yourself too seriously and that you should have all the fun you can. It will bring back those joyful feelings that are anchored to your artificial laugh.

The emphasis throughout this book is on enjoying life, getting rid of distress and having all the pleasure and fun you can while pursuing your goals and contributing to the world as much as possible. The theory is that by having fun, laughing and enjoying life, all will be well and you will experience the positive feelings of a good mental state. It's when you are unhappy and in a distressed state that I will start to worry about your mental health.

The Good Book of Godliness

Notes

The Good Book of Godliness

Notes

Chapter Thirteen

Meditate

Meditation will help you to contact God. To meditate you should close your eyes, clear your minds and try to have a positive attitude. Just allow thoughts to drift in and out of your mind but try not to think of any problems in your life.

Concentrate on your breathing. Allow a feeling of pleasantness and quietness to take over. Have a syllable or a word to repeat.

The word should have no meaning. A good word to use is "one" repeat it over and over, one, one, one, one. Concentrate on your breath coming in and out. Continue repeating your word and maintaining a passive peaceful attitude. Instead of repeating one word you could count to seven over and over or count to over, five of six over and over.

During meditation the sympallitic nervous system is not as active as at other times. You may feel calm and peaceful or happy. You

Chapter Thirteen
Meditate

should feel as if you are rising above the day to day routine and you should feel good. To get training in meditation you could go to a yoga training centre. Most of them have professionals who will guide you.

The Good Book of Godliness
Notes

Notes

Chapter Fourteen

Needs

Here are the needs that are important to all of us:

1. Love

2. Sex

3. Roof over your head

4. Food

5. Friends

6. The approval of others

7. Physical action

Unless these basic needs are satisfied we are likely to be unhappy.

Chapter Fourteen
Needs

Do a test on yourself and see if all of your needs are being met. If one or more of the categories are absent in your life, make a list of them.

Here are some suggestions to help you.

If love is what you are missing, think of the different ways you can receive love. The love of an animal is one of the nicest loves. Cats and dogs can be loving. Of the two cats are more independent as they don't need to be walked and will love you unconditionally. All you have to do is feed them, cuddle them and talk to them. They will do the rest. It makes coming home to an empty apartment or house, feel not so empty. Dogs require more attention as far as physical activity is concerned. So if you are in need of exercise and physical action, a dog is a good alternative that will fill several gaps in your life.

If sex is a problem, talk to your Doctor. There are many TV shows that talk about sexuality and living alone. One of the things they recommend is that you have a massage at least once a month. People need the physical touch, it doesn't have to be sex. If sex is what you need then try watching one of the many programs offered on TV.

Hopefully having a roof over your head is one of the things you need not put on your empty list, but if it is here are a few

Chapter Fourteen
Needs

suggestions. There are shelters available in every city – all you have to do is ask. Most churches or community centres will be able to help you.

Hopefully food is something that you are able to provide for yourself. If not the shelters and communities all have food drives.

If you are in need of friends, there are several ways you can go about meeting new people. The obvious is to join clubs or organizations. If money is an issue there are many free associations through your local church or YMCA. Volunteering is also a wonderful way to meet people that have the same interests as you. You can search either the computer or your local library for the different places that need volunteers. Here are a few suggestions: your local school; your church; community centre; help on an election or with a political party that is of interest to you; any of the non profit organizations would be thrilled to have a volunteer; Heart and Stroke, Cancer, Diabetes, just to name a few.

The Good Book of Godliness
Notes

Chapter Fifteen

Objectives

It is important that we have a purpose in life if we want to be happy. Our purpose could be to make the world a better place in which to live and to make other people happy. It doesn't have to be overwhelming, it could be simple like committing to recycle your garbage correctly.

Or it could be helping your community in cleaning the local park or planting trees. Another purpose could be to learn a new word every week and apply it to your work and social life. This objective would help not only in increasing your vocabulary but also is expanding your knowledge base.

Life should be a drive to help people but it should also be a drive to create something important.

If you have a worthwhile purpose and the ability to achieve that purpose you will likely be happy because you will always

Chapter Fifteen
Objectives

be working at something you like to do and you will get great satisfaction from achieving your goals.

There was a famous doctor who could have made a successful living as a pianist, or medical consultant but he preferred to spend his life in Africa helping underprivileged people.

The Good Book of Godliness
Notes

The Good Book of Godliness

Notes

Chapter Sixteen

Persistence

This is one of the secrets of success. The stories of great achievement where poor boys or girls rise to the top are nearly always backed up by persistence.

The person who thinks they may not make it and just keeps plugging ahead is usually the one who succeeds, he or she never thinks of failing they just keep trying and finally end up on top.

How do we get persistence? Often it is inherited or you may get it from your environment.

If your parents urge you to keep trying you may end up on top.

They say he never stopped trying. He never thought he could fail and he achieved his goal. It`s a part of your temperament. You may be born with it or it may develop in the early days of your life.

Chapter Sixteen
Persistence

If you find something you love to do and do it well you will be happy. Satisfaction from achievement will give you the power to keep plugging away until you achieve your goal.

The Good Book of Godliness

Notes

The Good Book of Godliness

Notes

Chapter Seventeen

Quiet

You have often heard it said that if you keep quiet the world will roll at your feet.

Listening is one of the best forms of communication.

Instead of talking, turn to listening. People like someone to listen to them. If you are a good listener, you will often persuade people to do things for you which they otherwise wouldn't do.

Listening is a powerful form of persuasion.

What do you really believe deep down? If you sit still and pray and meditate you can turn things around and get what you want.

Chapter Seventeen
Quiet

If God is with you , who can be against you? No matter what you are trying to do be sure you have God on your side. Pray, meditate, affirm, chant and listen to what your intuition is saying.

These techniques are often more persuasive then talking.

Notes

The Good Book of Godliness

Notes

Chapter Eighteen

Relax

Relaxation is essential to having a healthy outlook on life. Those who constantly rush and work under pressure bring stress and tension into their lives. Good performance at work cannot be achieved by people caught in a stressful cycle of tension and anxiety. Relaxation is the key to achieving your maximum potential. The day you learn to relax is the day you will find your right tempo and rhythm. You will then be calm, patient, and capable of managing with all that life deals you.

The relaxed person keeps in good physical condition and is patient and free of tension and distress. He remains cool, retains control, uses his head, and thinks clearly. He reads, studies, takes lessons, and uses every method to develop as a person. He shows initiative and has the vitality, energy and alertness to take on life's challenges.

Chapter Eighteen
Relax

I am going to show you how to relax generally so you will approach everything you do in life in a more effective manner. In this chapter I will give you specific working techniques, which will help you to relax and keep you cool under pressure. Let me show you some methods to help you get the maximum relaxation in your life. I suggest that you approach relaxing from three different directions:

1. Progressive relaxation

2. The Alexander method

3. A variety of interests.

Knowing how to relax requires knowledge of how tension and stress accumulate in the body and its muscles.

Because of the constant stimuli of radio, television, fast transportation, crowds of people, loud music, the excessive use of coffee, tea and alcohol, and lack of exercise and sleep, you are bombarded by a stream of noises, sights and artificial stimulation which can cause your muscles to become tense.

Dr. Edmund Jacobson, M.D. describes a technique of progressive relaxation in his book *You Must Relax*, 1976, New York: McGraw Hill. According to Dr. Jacobson, every time you use a muscle

Chapter Eighteen
Relax

in your arm or leg or finger, it is tensed by a message from your brain. When any muscle is extremely active, the nerve leading to that muscle is busy and using energy. If the muscles are kept in a constant state of tension, your energy is dissipated through overuse. Under continuing pressure, the muscles remain tense. This tension drains your energy, whether you are working or playing.

To get rid of this wasteful tension you must first recognize it. To do this, lie down flat on your back. Bend your right hand back at the wrist and hold it in this position until you get a feeling of tension in the muscle on the top side of your right arm, which is pulling your hand back. Make sure you feel this tension. Now let your hand drop forward and notice the tension disappear. Or has it completely disappeared? Maybe you can still feel some remaining tension in this muscle although it is not being actively used to move any part of your body.

This is wasteful tension and if you can recognize it, you may be able to get rid of it. Just let that part of your muscle go. Instead of tensing it, try to get it to do nothing, just the opposite of tension, until it becomes relaxed. Practice this for a few minutes.

Try bending our right hand forward at the wrist until you get the feeling of tension in the muscle on the underside of your arm. Now that you recognize it, try to get rid of this feeling of tension in that particular arm muscle by letting it go.

Chapter Eighteen
Relax

Lying flat on your back, pull the right forearm up to a vertical position by tensing the large muscle above the elbow. Now let your arm fall and try to let go completely and get the feeling that it is there, useless with no muscle supporting it. Practice this for a few minutes. Gradually you will start to develop the habit of relaxation in that large muscle.

Now try lifting up your entire right arm by the shoulder muscles to get the feeling of tension there. Then let your whole arm fall. Let these muscles go and try to get the feeling of relaxation in them. Practice this for a few minutes. Do this with the same muscles in the left arm. This relaxation can be extended to the leg by tensing and relaxing the various leg muscles in a similar manner.

Try to relax the muscles of the face and eyes. Put an exaggerated frown on your face with extra tension. Now relax the frown and try to get the feeling of relaxation in all the facial muscles. Next, close the eyes extremely tight, putting tension in the fine muscles around the eyes. Now open the eyes normally to get the opposite feeling of relaxation. Practice the same thing with the jaw. Grit your teeth and tighten your jaw with tension, then let your jaw fall open in a relaxed manner. You can do the same tensing and relaxing with the stomach muscles, the chest muscles and the back muscles.

Chapter Eighteen
Relax

Do all of these exercises several times, trying to get the feeling of tension, then of relaxation, throughout all the body muscles. End up in each case with a few minutes of complete relaxation of each set of muscles. Eventually your muscles will develop the habit of relaxing. As one muscle relaxes, it contributes to relaxation in all the others. So each time you get muscles into the habit of relaxing you are taking a step forward.

If you are finding it difficult to relax, you are probably not doing it right. You may be trying too hard and making too great an effort. Just try to let go. Relaxation is a condition in your muscles, which cannot be forced. It must come about naturally when the muscles let go. If you try to force a muscles to relax, you will build up more tension.

When you are completely relaxed you will have no feeling in your relaxed muscles. Every sensation goes away. You may not be able to feel your arms and legs. If you have any strong sensations you are not relaxing completely.

As you develop the habit of relaxing, you will become aware of any tension in your body and this will enable you to correct the wasting of energy it brings about. Relaxing will eventually become a reflex action, and when a muscle becomes tense it will automatically relax itself. The ideal you are aiming for is to have

Chapter Eighteen
Relax

the body automatically relax in every part when it is not being used for some particular purpose.

Nature's cure for tension is rest, but we frequently see people who get all the rest they want and still suffer from tension. When the muscles develop the habit and pattern of tension, it can take more than rest to cure this problem.

There are a number of theories on the best way to reduce muscle stress. F.M. Alexander developed a technique, which advocated re-aligning the body musculature so it will function as nature intended thereby relieving muscle stress, which can be the cause of a whole gamut of physical and psychic disorders.

The fascinating story of Alexander's' discovery of his technique, and the patience and dedication he brought to its development, is detailed in Sarah Barker's book, *The Alexander Technique: the Total Way to Body Health*.

Born in 1869 to a poor family in a remote outpost in the Australian bush country, Alexander was interested in the stage from the age of six. He began early in his life to give recitations and to work towards a career as an actor. However, he worked under a disability that proved to be the destiny factor in his life.

Chapter Eighteen
Relax

Sometimes during recitals his voice failed. The doctors whose advice he sought afforded him only temporary relief. One night, during an important engagement, he lost his voice completely and left the stage in despair.

Discouraged with the advice of doctors, Alexander began a close scrutiny of the way he used his body on stage, using mirrors as an aid for observation, to determine what had made him lose his voice. This enquiry led him beyond his immediate problem, and he became fascinated with the workings of the body, not only in speech, but during any physical activity. His findings evolved into the Alexander system of relaxation.

He realized that every movement he made was characterized by a tendency to pull his head backward and down. This was something he did when speaking in ordinary conversations, as well as during his stage appearances. It was more noticeable in formal recitation because there it produced a depression of the larynx and an audible sucking in of his breath. He discovered that pulling his head backward and down was part of a whole body pattern that included lifting his chest and hollowing his back, and this complex of body actions preceded every recitation he gave. When he stopped this negative action and started consciously to move his head and body upward, his voice disability was permanently corrected.

Chapter Eighteen
Relax

The philosophy behind the Alexander method is to move the body in a balanced and relaxed manner with only the effort absolutely necessary to complete a movement. Alexander felt the body should be used in such a way to allow it to perform at its maximum effectiveness. He claimed that when the body is held up straight, enough space is created within for the breath to massage the organs. Slumping or bending puts pressure on the organs so they are not able to perform well, and circulation slows down. He also claimed that unevenly stacked vertebrae in the spine caused pinching of nerves and lack of effectiveness in the parts of the body which they serve.

Alexander said the use of one basic movement to control all your body movements creates a relaxed condition throughout the body. He said the key to this smooth body control is the head and neck action, and he advocated letting the body's movements follow the upright action of the head.

When you are walking, gently move your head from side to side and up and down and let your head lead upward. This will straighten and relax the neck. Bringing your head into balance on top of your spine and letting your body follow its lead keeps the spine, bones and muscles in the body stacked in a way that allows the body to make smooth and balanced movements. Bend your head forward while moving it upward. Don't bend it backward.

Chapter Eighteen
Relax

Try to keep your head moving upward at all times. Even when you are lying in bed your head should be gently stretching upward toward the head of the bed to give you maximum relaxation. When sitting hold your head upward and the rest of your body will come into proper alignment and function in its most effective manner.

When walking, lift your legs from your hips and knees so you get the most efficient leverage in walking. Don't force your legs ahead, but rather lift them up from the hips and knees and put them down gently, this will enable you to walk with the least effort.

The human body is so constructed that when all the parts are balanced, it can stand erect and all the bones and ligaments are stacked in the right manner with the head leading at the top and everything else following. The body works efficiently with its energy going up through the body to the top. If you always move with the head leading upward so the head influences the movement of the body, all parts will work in harmony and you will notice a new efficiency in the way you relax and use your muscles.

If the head does not initiate your movements, the column of your body will not be stacked right and your muscles will not be coordinated. The result will be pressure on many body parts

Chapter Eighteen
Relax

due to excess muscular tension. In trying to control ourselves, we tend to pull our heads back and downward and shorten our necks, with our chests out and our backs arched. These tense habits make us feel that gravity is pulling us to pieces.

In order to follow the Alexander method, it isn't necessary to make any big aggressive movements of your head. The lengthening of your neck when you move your head upward is very small. Don't strain and push upward with a mighty effort. You don't have to stretch your neck like a giraffe. Just a slight upward movement of your head from the body is all that is required. Your body doesn't need to twist and turn to follow your head, but it just gently lengthens as your head is leading upward. This brings all the bones, vertebrae's and ligaments and muscles in your body into their natural alignment.

As you use the Alexander method you will feel more relaxed and natural and you will get a definite improvement in muscle tone, which will benefit your physical and mental health.

If you were to take a year off and just rest, go to bed early, sleep late, read, watch TV, putter in your garden, rest when you felt like it, and just generally relax and take things easy, you would be exhausted at the end of the year.

Chapter Eighteen
Relax

If you were to get into bed for the year and stay there all the time, having your meals served to you and just rest, sleep, read and watch TV, by the end of the year you would be dying. On the other hand, if you were to take a year off to write a book, sail your boat through the Caribbean, build yourself a house, head up a fund drive for your service club, take up a sport seriously or go back to university to take a course, at the end of the year you would be stimulated, energized and enthusiastic.

When you need a rest, you need a change. One way to relax and keep yourself in good mental condition is to get active in a variety of projects. Find the things you like to do, the things you do well and the things you feel proud of doing. Then get active in several fields of endeavor.

Study your life in the areas of family, social, education, hobbies, sports, social service, travel, and manual or mechanical activities to see if you can't bring a greater variety of interests into your life.

Variety of action and change of pace is what you need to help you relax. In addition to being more relaxed, you will be a more interesting person because of your varied interests. You will get along better with people, you will be wiser, and more creative, and you will have better mental health because mentally healthy

Chapter Eighteen
Relax

people are usually doing a wide range of things they do well, enjoy doing and feel good about.

You will have more energy because energy comes from doing interesting and exciting things. So search for areas of your life where you can win, achieve, create or develop your skills.

When you feel tense or under pressure while playing, push your head up with chin down and walk around gently. At the same time, breathe in to the count of seven and, breathe out to the count of seven. If you can also do your fake laugh ha, ha, ha, these things should relax you.

Don't forget your affirmation, which you can chant anytime to help you relax.

"I believe God is always within me, helping me to relax and giving me the strength to have fun. Thank you God."

The Good Book of Godliness

Notes

The Good Book of Godliness
Notes

Chapter Nineteen

Satisfaction

Are you satisfied with the way your life is going. Being satisfied will help you to get what you want Satisfaction from achievement is a powerful feeling.

If you are satisfied with the way your life is going you will be happy and positive.

Research has shown that people who laugh and enjoy life are more likely to succeed than grim, serious types, who don't enjoy life.

If you are satisfied with your life as it is, you will have the power to achieve more things.

Eustress is a form of stress which hits you when you do something well.

Chapter Nineteen
Satisfaction

Keep trying to get eustress in your life. How do you do it? Put your whole heart into what you are doing and do it well. This achievement will give you eustress.

The Good Book of Godliness

Notes

The Good Book of Godliness

Notes

Chapter Twenty

Tenacious

He or she never knows when they have achieved enough.

Tenacious is beyond persistence. Never say die. Keep on persisting and the result you want will likely appear.

Very successful people are usually tenacious. They keep plugging away. Never give up is their motto.

"If at first you don't succeed, try, try, again" is an affirmation which will help you.

If you can get your subconscious committed to this goal, you can't miss.

Nearly all great success stories are stories of tenacity.

Chapter Twenty
Tenacious

He or she never knew when to quit. They were beaten but they kept plugging and tenacity paid off.

If what you want isn't coming your way, stop, study, get more knowledge. Try in a different way.

These are the secrets of success.

Notes

The Good Book of Godliness

Notes

Chapter Twenty One

Understanding

Understanding is simply caring for the other person's viewpoint. It means considering all the problems that the other person has and giving him or her a fair chance to tell their stories.

It means looking into the other persons situation and giving them credit for doing as well as they are considering the adversities they are facing. It means trying to walk in the other persons shoes and see what it feels like to face all their adversities and to give consideration to their situation in your dealings with them

Understanding is usually a side effect of liking someone. If we like a person in our dealings with them we try to understand them and give them credit for what good things they are doing.

More knowledge will give you more understanding. If a person lets you down and fails to get result, try to find out why. When you find the reason for his failure you will have more understanding.

Chapter Twenty One
Understanding

Knowing the "why" behind what a person is doing will enable you to be more tolerant. You are likely to say "Now I know why he did that".

The more you know about the people involved the more you are likely to understand why they do or fail to do things.

The Good Book of Godliness

Notes

Notes

Chapter Twenty Two

Veracity

Veracity means telling it as it is and avoiding deceit and lying when making a deal. Veracity is honesty. It means facing the situation as it is and not twisting the facts.

It means the truth no matter how this goes against you. It means not exaggerating or boasting or blowing up the situation in your favour.

Veracity means being honorable and not taking advantage of your position to lie or do anything that will give you a benefit over your partner.

Sometimes you may lie or cheat to gain an advantage for yourself. It may work temporarily. However the truth may be some day revealed and you will be caught trying to cheat or get by trying to misrepresent the situation for your advantage.

Chapter Twenty Two
Veracity

The result could be catastrophic. Sometimes you may even to to jail and be required to spend many years behind bars because of what you did.

Generally speaking it doesn't pay to misrepresent a situation. The police are better equipped to deal with crime than you are to commit one.

The worst kind of crime (besides murder or rape) is the kind that you do that keeps you up at night! Think before you take action, it is so hard on your mind, body and soul to knowingly do something that is wrong. Many people have gone through life with terrible guilty consciences that has affected not only their relationships but their health as well.

Notes

The Good Book of Godliness

Notes

Chapter Twenty Three

Wisdom

Wisdom is certainly dependent on the quantity and quality of your knowledge. However you could have great knowledge but be lacking in wisdom.

How are you using the knowledge which you have? This will determine your wisdom.

You could have several university degrees and still be lacking in wisdom. We all know doctors and lawyers who have great knowledge but they don`t use it wisely.

Just sending a man to university won`t make him wise. We know of doctors and lawyers who are failing but have great knowledge. However more knowledge will usually help you to make wise decisions and increase your wisdom.

The Good Book of Godliness

Notes

Chapter Twenty Four

Youthful

This usually refers to those people who are under 20 years of age but sometimes we apply it to older ages.

You will often hear someone describe people in their sixties or seventies or even older as youthful in appearance.

What it usually means is that a person who keeps in excellent condition by dieting and exercising and having positive attitudes can look young. Sometimes a person with a positive life style who looks after their health can look youthful at ages fifty to seventy.

These people sometimes are referred to as youthful in appearance and attitude.

How do you maintain a youthful attitude and appearance? If you refer to my chapters on diet and meditating, these will guide you to have a happier, healthier life and you will be youthful.

The Good Book of Godliness
Notes

Chapter Twenty Five

Zen

I want to end this book with Zen.

Zen is part of Buddhism and means inner peace. Once you feel that you have inner peace it may be Zen. It can be used as a tool to persuade or relax.

I recommend using Zen when it is appropriate. If you don't understand something just assume that Zen will help you and keep persisting to get results.

It is in us all and up to us all to keep Zen where it belongs, without constantly struggling with it. If you don`t understand something just blame it on Zen and keep persisting to get results.

If you think of Zen as an attitude of mind it could bring Godliness into your life. You can use Zen in many ways. For example if you

Chapter Twenty Five
Zen

are upset or worried about something, call on Zen to soothe your mind.

There are many definitions of Zen. Here is one which I feel says it simply

ZEN: A school or division of Buddhism characterized by techniques designed to produce enlightenment. In particular, Zen emphasizes various sorts of meditative practices, which are supposed to lead the practitioner to a direct insight into the fundamental character of reality

The Good Book of Godliness

Notes